ARTHROSCOPIC ATLAS OF THE TEMPOROMANDIBULAR JOINT

David I. Blaustein DDS, PhD

Associate Professor and Former Head
Department of Oral and Maxillofacial Surgery
Director, Temporomandibular Joint and Facial Pain Clinic
College of Dentistry
University of Illinois at Chicago
Chicago, Illinois

Leslie B. Heffez DMD, MS, FRCD (c)

Associate Professor and Associate Head
Department of Oral and Maxillofacial Surgery
Temporomandibular Joint and Facial Pain Clinic
College of Dentistry
University of Illinois at Chicago
Chicago, Illinois

Lea & Febiger   Philadelphia • London • 1990

Lea & Febiger
600 Washington Square
Philadelphia, PA 19106-4198
U.S.A.
(215) 922-1330

Lea & Febiger (UK) Ltd.
145a Croydon Road
Beckenham, Kent BR3 3RB
U.K.

Library of Congress Cataloging-in-Publication Data

Blaustein, David I.
    Arthroscopic atlas of the temporomandibular joint / David
I. Blaustein, Leslie B. Heffez.
        p. cm.
    ISBN 0-8121-1242-3
    1. Temporomandibular joint—Examination—Atlases.   2.
Arthroscopy—Atlases.   I. Heffez, Leslie B.   II. Title.
    [DNLM: 1. Arthroscopy—atlases.   2. Temporomandibular
Joint—anatomy & histology—atlases.   3. Temporomandibular
Joint—physiology—atlases.   4. Temporomandibular Joint
Diseases—diagnosis—atlases. WU 17 B645a]
RK470.B53 1990
617.5′22—dc20
DNLM/DLC
for Library of Congress   89-13158
                                                                    CIP

Printed in the United States of America

Print Number 3   2   1

"The art of medicine consists of amusing the
patient while nature cures the disease."
Voltaire (1694–1778)

iii

ACKNOWLEDGMENTS

Samuel Collins' preparation of illustrative material for the chapters on arthroscopic anatomy is most gratefully acknowledged.

We are in deep gratitude to Nancy Novak for her tireless effort in preparing the photographs for the chapters on gross anatomy and arthroscopic instrumentation.

Our appreciation to Karl Storz Endoscopy-America, Inc. for supporting our initial efforts in this field and furnishing photographs of their equipment.

A special debt of gratitude to Stacy N. Heffez for her production of several key illustrations.

David I. Blaustein
Leslie B. Heffez

PREFACE

The *Arthroscopic Atlas of the Temporomandibular Joint* is a compilation of the research conducted and the experience gained at the University of Illinois at Chicago since September, 1983.

Our initial efforts in this field were directed toward examining the temporomandibular joints of embalmed cadaver specimens using the selfoscope endoscope. After much frustration and some gains, the acquisition of a rod lens telescope system allowed a major breakthrough. The increased image brightness and expanded field of view afforded by this instrument enabled us to make the detailed examinations on which this book is based.

Our experimental work moved, gradually, from the embalmed joint of a cadaver to that of the live baboon and then to the TMJ of a fresh cadaver. When we entered our first live human joint, it was with a confidence based on our experience in the dissecting laboratory and the animal operating room.

Immediately it was obvious that if we were to correctly interpret what we were seeing arthroscopically, correlations needed to be found with the well-established data provided by the imaging technologies. We were able to use many histologic specimens of both normal and abnormal TMJ's to confirm our arthroscopic impressions. Finally, given the limited area visible in any single arthroscopic view, a protocol for complete and systematic examination of the joint was needed.

This volume is organized to allow the reader to view the same kind of material that was the basis for our understanding of the arthroscopic anatomy and pathology of the TMJ.

We begin with chapters examining the gross and microscopic morphology and pathology of the joint. This material is presented as both a review and a constantly available reference for the reader moving through the succeeding chapters.

A section on arthroscopic technique and instrumentation precedes the chapters on arthroscopic anatomy and pathology. These latter chapters are profusely illustrated with color plates taken inside the TMJ. Each of these views is accompanied by a drawing of the plate. The relevant structures of these renderings are labeled, allowing us to leave the arthroscopic plates uncluttered. Imaging data (arthrotomograms and/or magnetic resonance images) are provided to document the accuracy of our arthroscopic interpretations.

In addition, we offer sections on problem solving and troubleshooting. The last chapter deals with problems of interpretation, intra- and postoperative complications, and instrument failure.

Finally, we include a glossary of arthroscopic terms in current use and a brief history of the discipline of endoscopy, with special emphasis on arthroscopy.

Arthroscopy of the TMJ is in its earliest stages. The basic equipment employed has been adapted from equipment commonly available to the orthopedist. We can look forward to alterations of equipment design more closely suited to our particular needs. Growth in interest and activity in TMJ arthroscopy has been explosive over the past years. Numerous continuing education courses have lately become available. Many clinicians register for multiple courses in hope of acquiring the basic knowledge necessary for the safe and effective use of TMJ arthroscopy. We hope that this volume will provide the clinician with a firm foundation from which learning and clinical experience can grow.

We believe that TMJ arthroscopy will radically alter the approach to diagnosis and management of TMJ dysfunction. The clinician might, however, be tempted to move ahead more rapidly than prudence, experience, and experimentally acquired data might dictate. We hope that such temptations will be resisted.

We encourage those of you who perform arthroscopic procedures on the TMJ to share your experience, through publication, with your colleagues. It is in the best interest of the patient, the arthroscopist, and the future of the discipline that the further development of TMJ arthroscopy proceed in accordance with, rather than in defiance of, the laws of logic and biology.

David I. Blaustein   Leslie B. Heffez
Chicago, Illinois

CONTENTS

NORMAL ANATOMY OF THE TEMPOROMANDIBULAR JOINT

1

The articulation of the human mandible with the cranium is a bilateral diarthrodial joint commonly known as the temporomandibular joint (TMJ) (Fig. 1-1). Anatomists use the term ginglymoarthrodial to describe the unique arrangement of bones forming both a hinge (*ginglymus*) and a sliding (*arthrodia*) joint. In the pure ginglymoid joint, a broad convex osseous structure fits into a corresponding concave osseous structure. The result is movement in one plane, as found in the elbow. In the pure arthrodia or *articulatio plana* the opposing osseous surfaces are nearly parallel. This results in the slight sliding or gliding motion seen in the intermetacarpal joints (Stedman's, 1982).

Each of the osseous components of the TMJ articulates with an interposed fibrous connective tissue disc (Figs. 1-2 and 1-3). Elsewhere in the body this relationship is found only in the acromioclavicular and sternoclavicular joints and the symphysis pubis (prior to fusion). This arrangement permits the range of motion unique to this joint (Warwick, Williams, 1968).

The anatomy of the adult temporomandibular joint is reviewed below. The muscles of mastication will not be discussed because they are not relevant to the development of an anatomic foundation for arthroscopy of the temporomandibular joint.

STRUCTURAL ANATOMY

OSSEOUS COMPONENTS

The craniad articulating surface is situated on the squamous part of the temporal bone anterior to the tympanic plate. Posteriorly, it consists of a concave articular fossa (*glenoid fossa*) and, more anteriorly, a convex *articular eminence* and *tubercle* contiguous with the somewhat flattened *infratemporal articulating surface* (usually described as part of the eminence) (Fig. 1-4) (Bhaskar, 1976, Oberg, Carlsson, 1979).

The glenoid fossa is concave in both the anteroposterior and mediolateral directions. It is bounded anteriorly, centrally, and medially by the articular eminence. Anterolaterally it is bounded by the articular tubercle, often described independently from the eminence. The tympanic plate of the temporal bone is its posterior boundary. This last structure is usually elongated inferiorly and posterolaterally into a variably prominent ridge called the *postglenoid tubercle*. Laterally, along its perimeter the articular fossa is bordered by a low ridge that is convex lateromedially. Medially, the fossa narrows and is bounded by a bony extension of the squamae of the temporal bone (Figs. 1-4 and 1-5). The bony fossa is divided into an anterior and posterior portion by a narrow slit, whose lateral extent is the *squamotympanic fissure* and whose medial extent is the *squamopetrous fissure*. Medially, the course of the squamotympanic fissure follows a triangular projection of the petrous portion of the temporal bone known as the *tegmen tympani*. The anterior extent of the tegmen tympani is bordered by the squamopetrous fissure and the posterior extent by the petrotympanic fissure (Figs. 1-4 and 1-5). The tegmen tympani does not form part of the articular component of the glenoid fossa. The squamotympanic fissure marks an approximate division of the fossa into articular and nonarticular portions, with articulation occurring anterior to this fissure (Oberg, Carlsson, 1979).

1

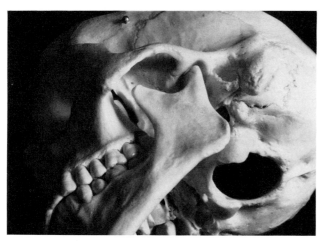

FIG. 1-1. Left temporomandibular joint, lateroinferior aspect. Note that the teeth are in occlusion. The apparent space between the mandibular condyle and glenoid fossa would be occupied by the condylar and glenoid fossa cartilages and articular disc.

The articular eminence consists of a transversely oriented bony ridge strongly convex in an antero-posterior direction and slightly concave in the mediolateral direction. Occasionally bony ridges mark the medial and lateral boundaries of the eminence (Figs. 1-4 to 1-6). The anterior extent of the eminence is contiguous with the infratemporal articulating surface (Fig. 1-7). This region is triangular with the base at the eminence and the apex oriented anteromedially. The orientation of the apex holds particular significance in arthroscopy of the superior joint space. This space is more limited lateroanteriorly than medioanteriorly. On the dried skull, the general extent of the infratemporal articulating surface may be inferred by the change in bony texture (Fig. 1-7) (Oberg, Carlsson, 1979).

The cephalad articulating surface is formed by the anterior and superior surfaces of the mandibular condyle (Fig. 1-8). The condyle is a semicylindric struc-

FIG. 1-2. Right TMJ in open position; normal condyle-disc-eminence relationship, sagittal microscopic section. Shrinkage of the specimen has caused the retrodiscal tissue (rdt) to lose its intimate relationship with the glenoid fossa. A flexure (fx) formed by the junction of the retrodiscal tissue and posterior band is seen. Note the position of the posterior band (pb), intermediate zone (iz), and anterior band (ab) of the disc. The anterior attachment (arrowheads) is formed of loose connective tissue with vascular elements. The articular surfaces of the eminence, glenoid fossa, and condyle are lined with fibrous connective tissue (arrows).

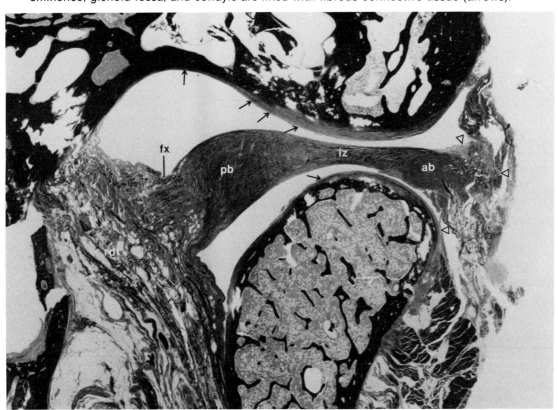

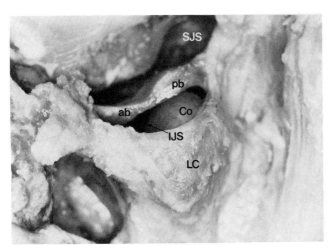

FIG. 1-3. Left TMJ; sagittal view of fresh cadaver dissection of a normal temporomandibular joint. The disc has been sectioned and partially excised to expose the inferior joint space (IJS) and superior joint space (SJS). The fibrous connective tissue covering of the condyle (Co) is intact. Note the morphology of the posterior band (pb), intermediate zone, and anterior band (ab). Only the inferior aspect of the lateral capsule (LC) is intact.

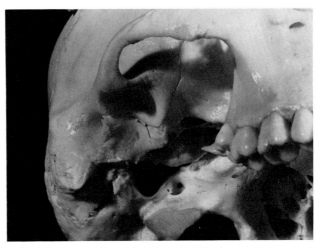

FIG. 1-5. The glenoid fossa and articular eminence, anteroinferior aspect. Note the prominence of the medial lip of the glenoid fossa. The tegmen tympani (arrow), bounded posteriorly by the petrotympanic fissure and anteriorly by the squamopetrous fissure, is indicated.

ture with its long axis running at approximately 90 degrees to the plane of the mandibular ramus (Fig. 1-9). Autopsy studies reveal mean condylar measurements of 20 mm mediolaterally and 10 mm anteroposteriorly, including the thickness of the soft tissues (Oberg et al., 1971). The degree of inclination (angulation) of the condyle is highly variable in the horizontal (Fig. 1-10) and vertical (Fig. 1-11) planes. The condyle (Fig. 1-12) is strongly convex anteroposteriorly and only slightly convex mediolaterally. Frequently, the mediolateral contour is found to be di-

FIG. 1-6. The temporomandibular joint, lateroanteroinferior aspect. Note the height and prominence of the articular eminence.

FIG. 1-4. The glenoid fossa, inferior aspect. Note the articular portion of the fossa anterior to the squamotympanic fissure (arrow).

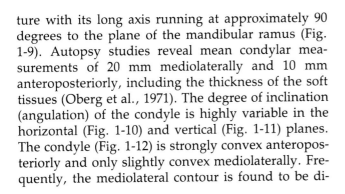

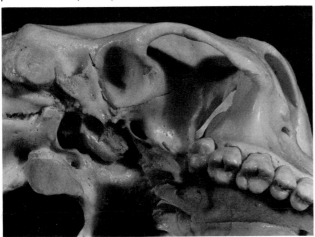

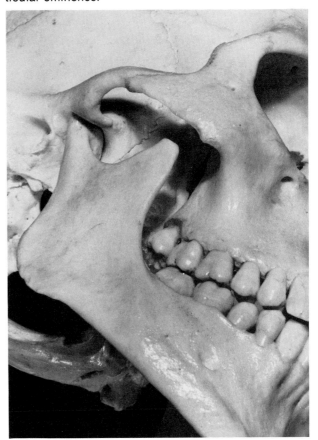

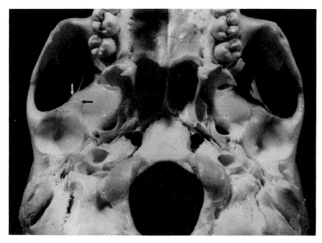

FIG. 1-7. The base of the skull. The outline of the infra-temporal articulating surface of the right temporal bone is indicated (arrows).

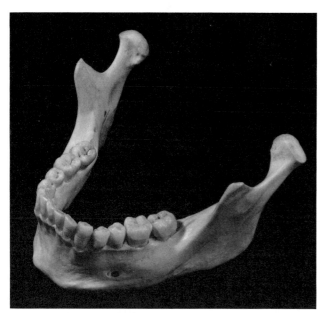

FIG. 1-8. The mandible, supero-oblique aspect. Note the angle formed by the long axis of the condylar head with the ramus.

FIG. 1-9. The mandible, superoposterior aspect.

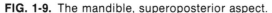
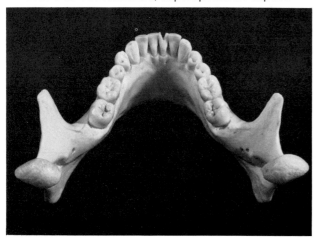

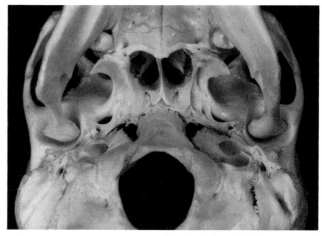

FIG. 1-10. The temporomandibular joint, inferior aspect. Note the horizontal angle formed by the condylar head and neck. Note also the apparent incongruity of the bony condyle and glenoid fossa. In the living patient, the articular disc and fossa and condylar cartilages correct this incongruity.

FIG. 1-11. The mandible, anterior aspect. Note the degree of vertical inclination (inclination viewed in the coronal plane) of the condyle.

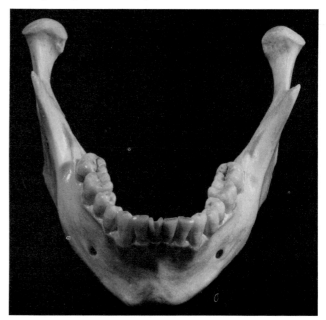

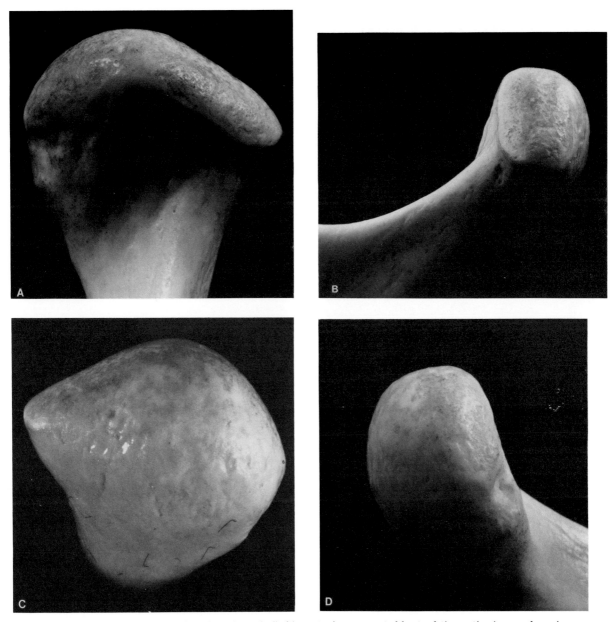

FIG. 1-12. *A*, Condylar head and neck (left), anterior aspect. Most of the articular surface is visible. *B*, The left condylar head, laterosuperior aspect. *C*, The left condylar head, posterosuperior aspect. *D*, The left condylar head, mediosuperior aspect.

vided into a medial and lateral portion by a sagittal crest. The lateral pole of the condyle is rather prominent, usually extending slightly lateral to the lateral surface of the mandibular ramus. The articulating portion of the condylar head is oriented superiorly and anteriorly. The inferior lamina of the retrodiscal tissue attaches along the posterosuperior aspect of the condyle. Frequently an osseous nutrient canal(s) may be visualized in this area on the dried skull (Bhaskar, 1976, Oberg, Carlsson, 1979).

ARTICULAR CARTILAGES

The articular surfaces of both the mandibular condyle and the glenoid fossa are covered by cartilage. This fibrocartilage differs from most other articular cartilage in the body by its surface layer of dense fibrous connective tissue (Figs. 1-2 and 1-13). In this way it most closely resembles the sternoclavicular and acromioclavicular joints. It is this fibrous connective tissue surface that interfaces directly with the fibrous

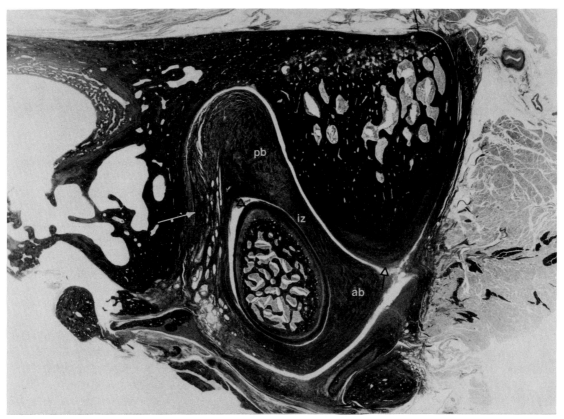

FIG. 1-13. Right TMJ; normal condyle-disc-fossa relationship, sagittal microscopic section, lateral condylar region. The fibrous connective tissue covering of the eminence and condyle are particularly evident (open arrows). Note the fibrous connective tissue disc: posterior band (pb), intermediate zone (iz), and anterior band (ab). The retrodiscal tissue (arrow) is collapsed in the closed position.

connective tissue intra-articular disc on its craniad and cephalad surfaces.

Microscopically, six tissue layers are identified in the condyle and temporal bone; named from the joint cavity inward, they are (1) fibrous connective tissue covering, (2) undifferentiated fibroblasts (proliferative layer), (3) intermediate layer, (4) cartilage, (5) compact bone, and (6) spongy bone. There are regional differences in the thickness and composition of each of these layers, perhaps due to differential growth rates and functional load (Oberg, Carlsson, 1979). For example, the fibrous connective tissue layer of the posterior slope of the articular tubercle is thick enough to be arranged in two definite layers with an intermediary transitional zone (Bhaskar, 1976).

CAPSULE AND LIGAMENTS

The capsule is attached superiorly to the circumference of the articular fossa and the articular eminence. Inferiorly it is attached to the neck of the man-

dibular condyle and to the disc, separating the joint cavity into two compartments. The joint capsule is described as having two components: an outer fibrous capsule, the *stratum fibrosum*, which fuses with the ligaments; and an inner synovium, the *stratum synovium*. The TMJ is enclosed by a connective tissue capsule reinforced by ligaments except for its anteromedial two thirds. The horizontal fibers of the external pterygoid muscle reinforce the anteromedial parts of the capsule (Oberg, Carlsson, 1979, Mahan, 1980).

The synovium consists of an intimal layer resting on a vascular connective tissue known as the subintima. The intima is rich in cells and thin-walled vessels, in contrast to the subintima, which is predominantly fibrous. The fiber arrangement and thin-walled vascular spaces of this structure, best seen in sagittal microscopic sections, permit a wide range of mandibular motion (Fig. 1-14). Only the nonload-bearing surfaces of the TMJ are lined with synovium. In the region of the squamotympanic fissure and eminence, there is a reflection or extension of synovium

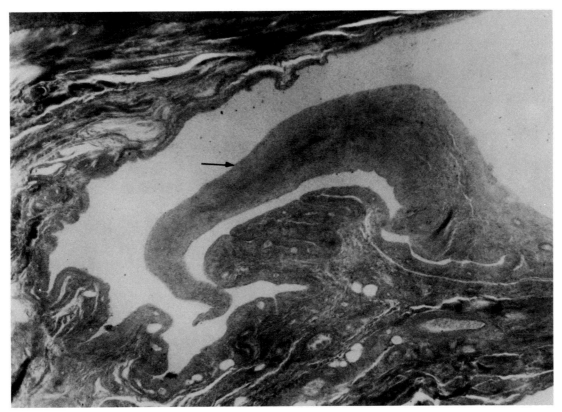

FIG. 1-14. Sagittal microscopic section (100 X). Note the synovial plica (arrow) with connective tissue and vascular core.

covering the retrodiscal tissue and anterior attachment, respectively. In addition, the posterior and anterior recesses of the inferior joint space have a well-defined synovial membrane (Griffin, Sharpe, 1960a,b). The larger vessels of the synovium are typically seen to lie transversely and are readily observed during arthroscopy (see Chapter 4).

The intimal layer is typical of the intima of other synovial joints and functions to augment the constituents of the synovial fluid by producing certain of its components. Normal synovial fluid consists of a hyaluronic acid–protein complex with little or no sulfated glycosaminoglycans (GAGs). It is generally considered a blood plasma dialysate (Lever, 1958). Also, the intima functions to selectively filter, by molecular weight, elements entering the joint space by way of the blood. Phagocytes within the intima are capable of removing certain materials from the joint space. (Oberg, Carlsson, 1979) Synovial fluid in itself may act as a buffer against compressive loading forces (Macconail, 1950).

Ligaments are, essentially, fibrous connective tissue condensations of the capsule. Functionally the ligaments protect the joint by maintaining stability, especially in the mediolateral direction, influencing the movements of opposing joint surfaces, and guiding the joint surfaces into the proper relationship for optimum function (Harty, 1984).

Laterally, the capsule is reinforced by several thickenings, termed variously the *temporomandibular ligament, lateral ligament,* or *lateral temporomandibular ligament.* The principal band of this ligament runs an oblique course downward and backward from the lateral surface of the zygomatic arch to the posterior border of the condylar neck. A second, more deeply situated band is also present, with fibers running in a somewhat more horizontal direction. This fibrous connective tissue band also originates from the lateral surface of the zygomatic arch; however, it terminates on the condylar neck slightly anterior to its obliquely oriented counterpart (Rees, 1954, Oberg, Carlsson, 1979).

The structure known as the *medial capsular ligament* is a thickening of the posterior one half to two thirds of the medial capsule (Warwick, Williams, 1980). This ligament is not as thick as the lateral ligament and is formed by a single band of fibers generally oriented anterosuperior to posteroinferior (Oberg and Carlsson, 1979). Its anterior extent is slightly thickened and abruptly terminates, leaving the remaining medial

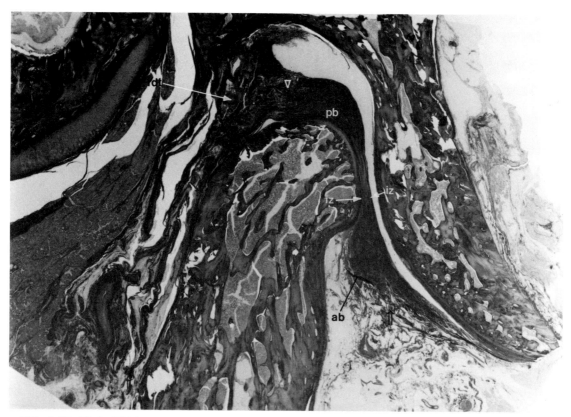

FIG. 1-15. Right TMJ, normal condyle-disc-fossa relationship, sagittal microscopic section, mid-condylar region. Note the intra-articular components from posterior to anterior: retrodiscal tissue (rdt), posterior attachment (arrowhead), posterior band (pb), intermediate zone (iz), anterior band (ab), and anterior attachment (double arrow).

capsule unsupported (Rees, 1954, Mahan, 1980). We will show in Chapters 5 and 6 that this abrupt ligamentous termination is an important arthroscopic landmark (Heffez, Blaustein, 1987, Blaustein, Heffez, 1988).

Two additional, or accessory, ligaments may play a role in the function of the temporomandibular joint: the *sphenomandibular* and *stylomandibular ligaments*. These ligaments may protect the joint in wide excursive movements, even though they are not intimately associated with the articulation. The sphenomandibular ligament is a flat band of fibrous connective tissue attached superiorly to the angular spine of the sphenoid bone. It descends and inserts inferiorly on the lingula of the mandibular foramen. The stylomandibular ligament is a specialized band of cervical fascia extending from the tip of the styloid process of the temporal bone to the angle and posterior border of the mandibular ramus (Warwick, Williams, 1980, Mahan, 1980).

THE DISC AND ITS ATTACHMENTS

The intra-articular tissue consists of several named parts, only certain of which can be described as "disc"

proper. From posterior to anterior, the intra-articular tissue has been divided into the retrodiscal tissue (superior lamina craniad and inferior lamina cephalad),

FIG. 1-16. Sagittal view of fresh cadaver dissection of a normal right TMJ. The lateral capsule has not been dissected from the lateral pole of the condyle. The superior joint space (SJS) is seen. Note the upward bulge of the posterior band (arrow) and intermediate zone (arrowhead). The photograph suggests a retrodiscal tissue (open arrows) that differs from that of the posterior band.

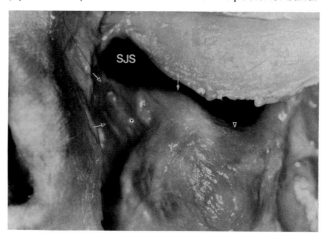

including the posterior attachment; the disc, including the posterior band, intermediate zone (central zone), and anterior band; and finally the anterior attachment (Rees, 1954), (Figs. 1-2 and 1-15). Additional subdivisions have been named to describe the structures resulting from the pathologic remodeling that occurs with internal derangements (see Chapters 2 and 6). The term "disc," rather than "meniscus," is used here because meniscus more appropriately describes crescent-shaped, fibrous structures that are lenticular in shape (Stedman's, 1982).

The fibrous connective tissue articular disc is interposed between the articular surfaces. The disc, along with its attachments, completely separates the joint space into two synovium-lined cavities named the superior joint space (or *temporodiscal*) and the inferior joint space (or *condylodiscal*) (Figs. 1-16 to 1-19) (Oberg, Carlsson, 1979, Mahan, 1980).

The superior joint space is bounded superiorly by the connective tissue covering the glenoid fossa, eminence, and infratemporal articulating surface, and inferiorly by the superior surface of the retrodiscal tissue and disc (Figs. 1-2 and 1-18). The inferior space is bounded superiorly by the disc and retrodiscal tissue, and inferiorly by the fibrous connective tissue covering the cartilage of the condyle (Figs. 1-2, 1-18 and 1-19). The volumes of both the superior and inferior joint spaces have been measured on cadaver

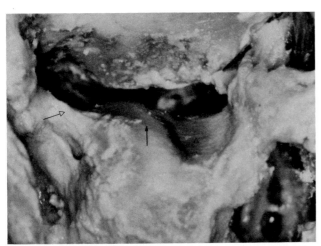

FIG. 1-17. Sagittal view of fresh cadaver dissection of a normal right TMJ. The lateral aspect of the glenoid fossa and eminence have been drilled away to expose the superior surface of the disc. Note the retrodiscal tissue (open arrow), posterior band (arrow), and intermediate zone (arrowhead).

FIG. 1-18. Sagittal view of fresh cadaver dissection of a normal right TMJ. The disc has been sectioned and the lateral portion removed, exposing the inferior joint space (IJS). Note the fibrous connective tissue covering of the condyle (Co). The posterior band (pb), intermediate zone (iz), and anterior band (ab) of the disc are visible.

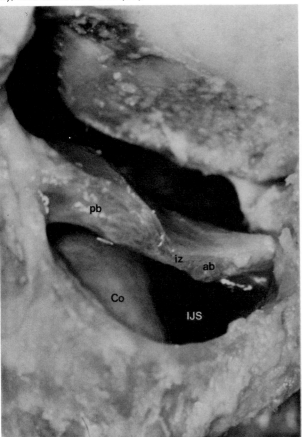

FIG. 1-19. Sagittal view of fresh cadaver dissection of a normal right TMJ. The medial half of the disc (arrows) is elevated superiorly to expose the inferior joint space and condyle (Co).

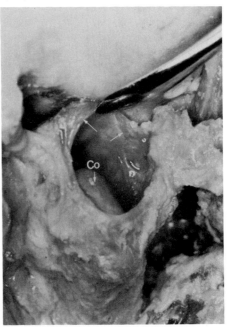

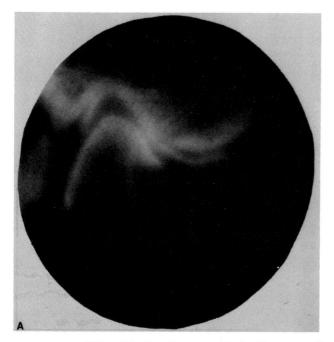 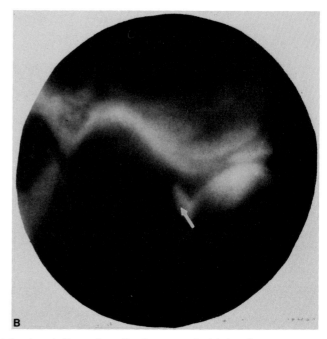

FIG. 1-20. Single-contrast, double-compartment horizontally and vertically corrected lateral cephalometric arthrotomograms. Normal right TMJ in closed (*A*) and open (*B*) positions. Minimal dye has been injected to opacify the joint spaces. The disc is represented by the radiolucent biconcave structure. Note that the junction of the retrodiscal tissue and posterior band cannot be precisely determined with this technique. This junction is suggested in the open position (*B*) when the dye in the posterior recess of the inferior joint space is deflected superiorly (arrow).

specimens (Toller, 1974). On this basis, the superior joint space has been described as having a mean volume of 1.2 ml and the inferior joint space a mean volume of 0.9 ml. Experience with arthrography suggests that much smaller volumes exist: 0.4 to 0.5 ml and 0.2 to 0.3 ml for superior and inferior spaces, respectively (Fig. 1-20A, B). Observations made from magnetic resonance imaging (MRI) suggest that the spaces are virtual, with the signal intensity of synovial fluid being difficult to identify (Fig. 1-21A, B).

The gross structure of the normal disc is biconcave and completely fills the joint cavity, providing only a potential space between it and the articular surfaces. The disc is attached medially and laterally to the condylar head, where it forms a junction with the medial

and lateral walls of the capsule and its ligaments. These junctions form recesses or fornices. Posteriorly, the disc is attached to the temporal bone superiorly, and the condylar neck inferiorly via the retrodiscal tissue (bilaminar zone) (Rees, 1954). Anteriorly the picture is less clear, with the disc apparently merging with the anterior and anteromedial parts of the capsule and attaching to the anterior margin of the eminence above and the anterior articular margin of the condyle below (Figs. 1-22, 1-23 and 1-24) (Rees, 1954).

The disc proper consists of three transversally ellipsoid regions: *anterior band, intermediate zone,* and *posterior band,* measuring a mean 2.0, 1.1, and 2.8 mm, respectively (Figs. 1-2 and 1-15) (Rees, 1954, Hansson et al., 1977). These components have in common

→

FIG. 1-21. Parasagittal T_1-weighted (TR 800; TE 20 msec) magnetic resonance image of normal left TMJ, in closed (*A*) and open (*B*) positions, obtained with surface coil. *A*, Note the low signal intensity of the normal disc (open arrow). The posterior band is not clearly defined. The retrodiscal tissue (arrow) displays a homogenous, intermediate signal intensity. Cortical bone of the glenoid fossa and eminence (arrowheads) and condyle (double arrow), and air in the ear canal (eac) display various low signal intensities. Blood within fast-flowing vessels (bv) demonstrates the signal void phenomenon. The fatty marrow (*) within the adult condyle has a high signal intensity. *B*, Note how the retrodiscal tissue (rdt) hugs the roof of the glenoid fossa (series of arrows) and displays a heterogenous signal of low and intermediate intensities. The low signal intensity of the normal disc (open arrows) can also be noted.

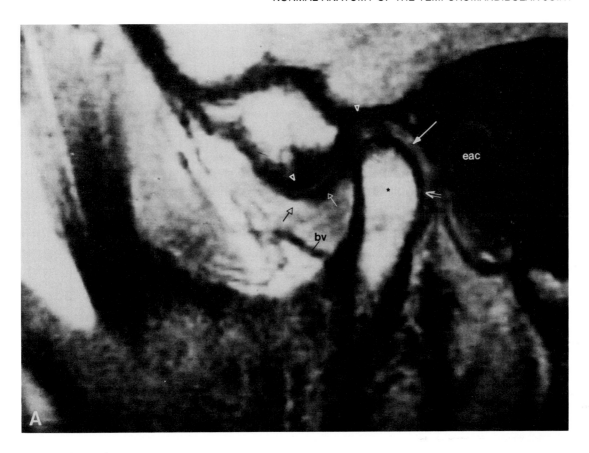

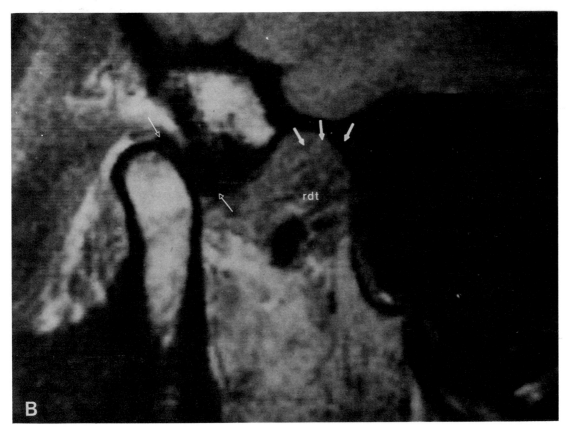

dense fibrous connective tissue as their main structural component. The actual boundaries between these components are not readily apparent. The internal architectural pattern of the fibrous connective tissue can be used to identify the disc components (Strauss et al., 1960, Scapino, 1984). The anterior and posterior bands contain fibers that run both anteroposteriorly and mediolaterally. Vertically oriented fibers (that is, oriented at right angles to the disc surface) also have been found in the posterior band (Scapino, 1984). The collagen fiber organizational patterns in each of these disc parts is probably functional (Figs. 1-2 and 1-25). Few elongated fibroblasts are found within the disc. The fibrous nature and limited vascularity of the disc suggest limited reparative ability. In the adult, some fibroblasts may differentiate into chondroid cells and eventually true chondrocytes. Rarely, islands of hyaline cartilage may be identified within the disc. These cellular changes appear to depend on mechanical loading (Bhaskar, 1976).

The attachments of the disc to the retrodiscal tissue (posterior attachment) and anterior capsule (anterior attachment) are not distinct. Posteriorly a short knife-edged prolongation of the synovium of the posterior attachment is present over the superior surface of the posterior band (Fig. 1-26). More deeply at the junction of the posterior band and the posterior attachment is a transitional area where the internal architectural pattern of the fibrous connective tissue becomes dense and less random, with some vascular elements (Fig. 1-2). The anterior and posterior attachments increase in vascularity as they approach their junctions with the capsule at the periphery of the joint. The anterior attachment changes from a relatively dense fibrous connective tissue to an apparently areolar type as it attaches to the anterior capsular wall (Fig. 1-2). The posterior attachment likewise increases markedly in vascularity and neural content posteriorly. It ultimately forms the highly vascular *retrodiscal tissue* (Figs 1-2 and 1-24). This structure has been described as having a superior elastic component and inferior collagenous component with an interposing

FIG. 1-22. Normal sagittal microscopic section; mid-condylar region. Note the flexure (fx). The arthroscopist usually performs the diagnostic examination with the mandible approximating the semi-open position, as seen here. Note the bilaminar arrangement of the retrodiscal tissue. The fibrous inferior lamina (arrowheads), vascular mid-region, and elastic superior lamina (arrow) may be seen.

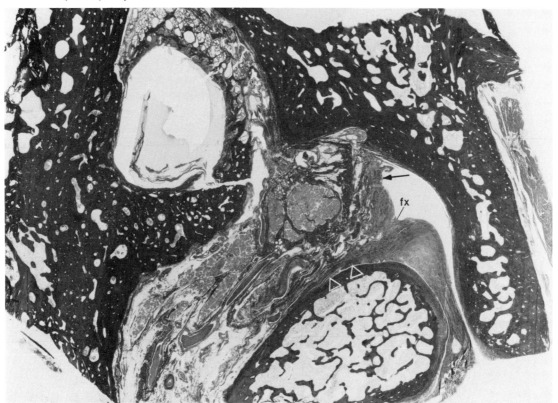

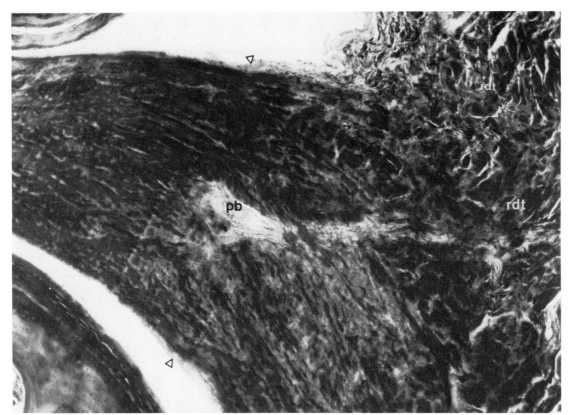

FIG. 1-23. Sagittal microscopic section of the posterior band (pb) and retrodiscal tissue (rdt) (100 ×); mid-condylar region, normal condyle disc-fossa relationship. Note the vascular elements within the retrodiscal tissue. The synovial membrane (arrowheads) can be seen extending onto the superior and inferior aspects of the disc.

neurovascular connective tissue zone (Rees, 1954, Griffin, 1959). The superior stratum attaches to the squamotympanic fissure, and the inferior stratum to the inferior margin of the posterior articular slope of the condyle (Griffin, Sharpe, 1960a). Rees (1954) demonstrated the extensibility of this tissue as ranging from 7 to 10 mm in the fresh cadaver specimen.

We described the junction of the posterior band of the disc and the temporal attachment of the retrodiscal tissue as the **flexure** (Figs. 1-2, 1-22, and 1-26), (Heffez, Blaustein, 1987). Topographically, the posterior band is oriented horizontally or slightly anterosuperiorly at this junction, and the temporal lamina of the bilaminar zone of the retrodiscal tissue is oriented posterosuperiorly, forming a U or V (Heffez, Blaustein, 1987). (This topographic arrangement will be discussed in greater detail in Chapter 5.)

The retrodiscal tissue consists of loose fibrous connective tissue of the areolar type interspersed with large venous sinuses and numerous small arteries and arterioles. The endothelial lined spaces (sinuses) are collapsed in the closed-jaw (retruded condyle) po-

sition. They expand as the condylar head and articular disc become positioned anteriorly in the translational phase of jaw opening. In this situation, the retrodiscal tissue hugs the glenoid fossa and posterior aspect of the condyle (Fig. 1-21). The initial filling of the retrodiscal tissue plexus may be due, in part, to the creation of a negative pressure in the vascular spaces. When the jaw is opened, the shape of the vascular retrodiscal tissue is "fan-like" in sagittal view. As the jaw closes, the retrodiscal tissue decreases markedly in volume as the blood is forced out of the sinuses. MR imaging demonstrates this situation well (Fig. 1-21). The expansion of retrodiscal tissue is maintained with prolonged opening, indicating that additional factors may operate. The presence of *"sperrarterien,"* as is found in the lung, kidney, and vertebral venous plexuses, may be a significant factor in the ability of the retrodiscal plexus to empty and refill with each masticatory cycle (Griffin, 1959, Le Gros Clark, 1958). Nerves are usually seen close to the arteriovenous anastomoses (Griffin, Sharpe, 1960a). The stretching and distortion of the connec-

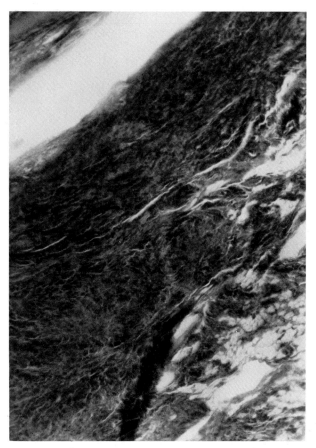

FIG. 1-24. Sagittal microscopic section of the anterior attachment (100X); mid-condylar region, normal condyle-disc-fossa relationship. To the right is anterior. This structure is characterized by loose connective tissue with vascular elements, though the vessels are less abundant than in the retrodiscal tissue.

tive tissue elements in the retrodiscal tissue may also assist in the expansion of collapsed blood vessels.

FUNCTIONAL ANATOMY

The retrodiscal pump provides an abundant and ever-changing supply of blood to the joint cavity. One possible function of this constant replenishment of blood might be to contribute to the blood-filtrate component of the synovial fluid (Griffin, 1959). An interesting hypothesis suggests that this rapidly changing vascular pool provides an ever-present new source of cartilage-nourishing elements to the synovial fluid, with the *pump* compensating for the relatively low ratio of synovial fluid:cartilage in this joint (Le Gros Clark, 1958, Griffin, 1959). Furthermore, Adkins, Davies (1940) observed that absorption from synovial cavities was significantly accelerated by movement.

As the metabolic activity of synovial cavities is cyclic and intermittent, a vascular pump mechanism might be required for replenishment of nutrients.

MOVEMENT

During the earliest (rotational) stage of the opening movement, the condyles rotate about a stationary bi-condylar axis and the posterior aspect of the condyle is brought into closer relationship with the posterior band. As opening progresses, the bicondylar axis moves forward and downward, while at the same time, the condyle rotates about this axis down the inclined plane of the intermediate zone. In the later stages of opening, the condyle-intermediate zone complex moves down the posterior slope of the articular eminence. The extent of forward movement is limited by the polar attachments of the disc, the posterior tympanic attachment of the retrodiscal tissue, and the lateral temporomandibular ligament. The inextensible inferior stratum of the retrodiscal tissue assists in translatory and hinge movements when the superior stratum is taut. The retrodiscal tissue moves inward to fill the void created by the translation of the disc. The posterior band now lies in a posterior relation to the condylar head. Different parts of the disc are interposed between condyle/glenoid fossa or eminence in different jaw positions. During translation, the excursion of the condyle is greater than the excursion of the disc because of relative movements between condyle and disc. In the *normal* joint, both hinge and translatory movements occur within the lower compartment; only translatory movements occur in the superior compartment (Rees, 1954).

Anterior and posterior movement movement of the articular disc has been ascribed to a number of factors, ranging from anterior traction by the superior head of the external pterygoid muscle (anterior movement) (Mahan, 1980) to elastic recoil of the superior stratum and relative inextensibility of the inferior stratum of the retrodiscal tissue (posterior movement) (Rees, 1954). Carpentier et al. (1988) have shown that the majority of fibers of the superior head of the lateral pterygoid muscle merge with those of the inferior head to insert on the condyle. Only a few fibers insert onto the disc, and these are found only on its medial aspect. These fibers are occasionally visible on arthroscopy through the medial capsule (Chapter 5). Several authors have investigated the function of the superior and inferior heads of the external pterygoid muscle using electromyography and concluded that the two parts of the muscle functioned independently (Kamiyama, 1961, McNamara, 1973). McNamara

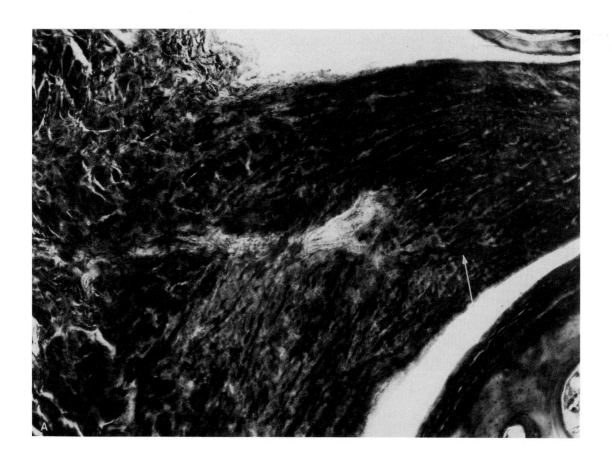

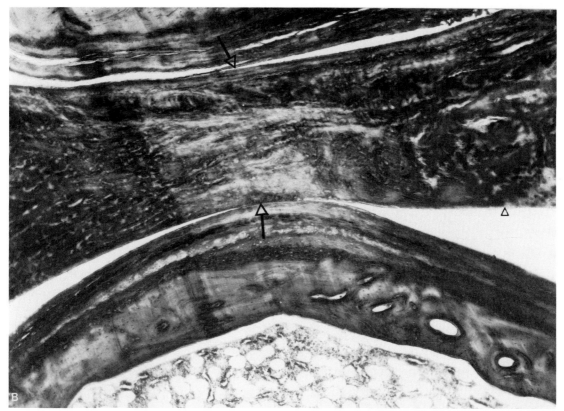

FIG. 1-25. *A* and *B*, Composite sagittal microscopic sections of the disc (100 ×) demonstrating the fiber architecture of the posterior band (arrow), intermediate zone (open arrows), and anterior band (arrowhead).

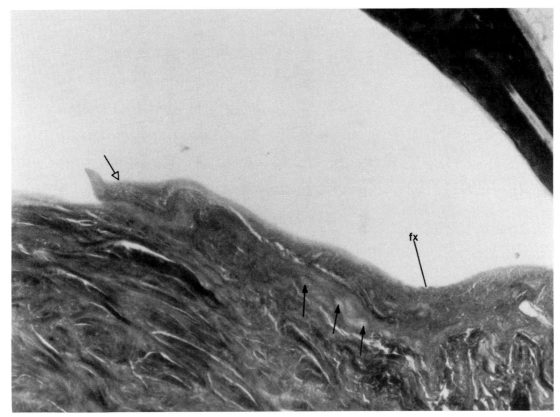

FIG. 1-26. The knife-edged prolongation of the synovium covering the posterior attachment (open arrow) over the posterior surface of the posterior band contains few transverse vessels (arrows). In the normal disc position, this structure never extends beyond the crest of the posterior band. Note the flexure (fx).

(1973) postulated that the role of the superior head was to stabilize the condyle and disc during closing movements and that the inferior head assisted in translation. The most plausible explanation for co-ordinated condyle-disc movement would involve generation of a shear force by the condyle against the anterior band and intermediate zone.

CONDYLE RELATIONSHIPS

In the sagittal anatomy of the *normal* joint, the posterior band occupies the area of maximum concavity of the articular fossa. The rapidly thinning anterior extent of this tissue (intermediate zone) lies along the posterior slope (incline) of the articular eminence. At this site, the internal architecture of the collagen fibers changes abruptly, with most fibers now oriented anteroposteriorly (Figs. 1-2 and 1-22, 1-25). The intermediate zone expands anteriorly and inferiorly into the anterior band that underlies the infratemporal articulating surface (Figs. 1-15 and 1-18).

The disc thickening known as the posterior band lies at an approximately 12:00 to 1:00 o'clock position with respect to the condylar head (Fig. 1-15). The relationship of the intermediate zone to the eminence and condyle has been determined mathematically from horizontally and vertically corrected arthrotomograms (Heffez et al., 1988). This method is illustrated in Figure 1-27. The slightly forward tilting slope of the anterior surface of the condylar head is in relation to the most anterior part of the posterior band and the most posterior part of the intermediate zone when the jaw is closed. The distribution of glycosaminoglycans (GAGs) suggests that these areas are load bearing (Kopp, 1976). Kempson et al., (1970) noted the occurrence of GAGs in tissue exposed to load. The GAGs increase resistance to compression by imbibing and retaining water by osmosis (Kopp, 1978). The predilection of the sulfated GAGs for the lateral part of the temporal eminence and anterior portion of the condyle concurs with the current presumptions about TMJ loading. We will see later, that in internal derangements, greater remodeling

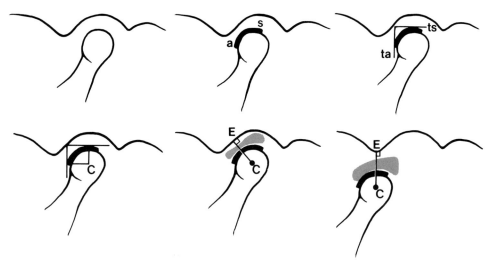

FIG. 1-27. Illustration demonstrating method for describing the position of the thin zone (intermediate zone) of the disc. Row 1 (left to right): Tangents (ts, ta) are drawn at the points of minimal (superior point) (s) and maximal (anterior) (a) sectional curvatures of the condyle. Row 2 (left to right): The center of the working surface of the condyle is then located by dropping perpendiculars from the tangents. The thin zone is located along the mechanical center of the joint, that is, along a perpendicular drawn from the center of the working surface of the condyle (C) to the posterior slope of the eminence (E).

changes are noted laterally on arthroscopy, offering additional support to the argument that the medial aspect of the temporal bone is relatively unloaded.

Knowledge of the anatomic relationships of the joint components is essential to carrying out successful diagnostic arthroscopy. Thorough familiarity with both the static and dynamic morphology of the joint is imperative. Equally important is a knowledge of the color, surface morphology, texture, orientation of structures, joint space configuration, and topographic relationships. While these areas will be discussed at length in Chapters 2, 5, and 6, the surface vascular patterns of the normal retrodiscal tissue, disc, and synovium should be mentioned here. We will be speaking in terms of relative vascularity as viewed grossly and topographically, rather than histologically. The surface vascularity may not accurately reflect the underlying histologic structure. We have found that establishing the presence or absence of surface vascularity is crucial to diagnostic arthroscopy. The disc is avascular and appears stark-white. The retrodiscal tissue may contain several surface vessels and certainly many deeper vessels; hence its pink color. The thin prolongation of the synovium of the posterior attachment over the posterior band contains a few surface vessels and should not be thought of as pathologic (Fig. 1-23). A few synovial vessels may be noted where the synovium merges with the disc within the capsular sulci. The concept of surface vascularity will be treated in much greater depth in later

chapters (Heffez, Blaustein, 1987, Blaustein, Heffez, 1988).

REFERENCES

Adkins EWO, Davies DV: Absorption from the joint cavity. Quart J Exp Physio 30, p. 1940.

Bhaskar SN ed; *Orban's Oral Histology and Embryology*. St Louis, CV Mosby Co, 1976, pp 395–404.

Blaustein DI, Heffez L: Diagnostic arthroscopy of the temporomandibular joint. Part II: Pathological arthroscopic findings. Oral Surg 66(2):135–141, 1988.

Carpentier P, Yung JP, Marguelles-Bonnet R et al. Insertions of the lateral pterygoid muscle: An anatomic study of the human temporomandibular joint. J Oral Maxillofac Surg 46:477–482, 1988.

Griffin CJ: Mechanism of blood supply to the synovial membrane. Aust Dent J 4:379–384, 1959.

Griffin CJ, Sharpe CJ: The structure of the human temporomandibular meniscus. Aust Dent J 5:190–199, 1960a.

Griffin CJ, Sharpe CJ: The distribution of the synovial membrane and the mechanism of its blood supply in the adult human temporomandibular joint. Aust Dent J 5:367–372, 1960b.

Hansson T, Oberg T, Carlsson GE, et al.: Thickness of the soft tissue layers and the articular disk in the temporomandibular joint. Acta Odontol Scand 35:77, 1977.

Harty M: Knee Joint Anatomy. In Arthroscopy: Diagnostic and Surgical Practice, Casscells, SW (Ed.) Philadelphia, Lea & Febiger 1984, pp. 3–9.

Heffez L, Blaustein DI: Diagnostic arthroscopy of the temporomandibular joint. Part 1: Normal arthroscopic findings. Oral Surg 64(6): 653–678, 1987.

Heffez L, Jordan S, Going R: Determination of the radiographic position of the temporomandibular joint disk. Oral Surg 65(3):272–280, 1988.

Kamaiyama T: An electromyographic study on the function of the external pterygoid muscle. Bull Tokyo Med Dent Univ 8:118, 1961.

Kempson GE, Muir H, Swanson SAV, et al.: Correlations between stiffness and the chemical constituents of cartilage on the human femoral head. Biochemica & Biophysica Acta 215:70–77, 1970.

Kopp S: Topographical distribution of sulfated glycosaminoglycans in human temporomandibular joint disks. A histochemical study of autopsy material. J Oral Path 5:265–276, 1976.

Le Gros Clark WE: *The Tissues of the Body*. 9th ed, Oxford, Clarendon Press 1958.

Lever JD, Ford EHR: Histological, histochemical and electron microscoipic observation on the synovial membrane. Anat Rec 123(4):525–539, 1958.

MacConail MA: The movements of bones and joints. The synovial fluid and its assistants. J Bone & Joint Surg, 32B, 244–252, 1950.

Mahan P In Irby WB (eds): *Current Advances in Oral Surgery.* Vol III St Louis, CV Mosby Co, 1980, pp. 3–9.

McNamara JA Jr: The independent functions of the two heads of the lateral pterygoid muscle. Am J Anat 138:197, 1973.

Oberg T, Carlsson GE, Fajers CM: The tempormandibular joint. A morphological study on a human autopsy material. Acta Odontol Scand 29:349, 1971.

Oberg T, Carlsson GE: In Zarb GA, Carlsson GE: *Temporomandibular Joint Function and Dysfunction.* Copenhagen, Munksgaard, 1979, pp 101–118.

Rees LA: The structure and function of the mandibular joint. Br Dent J 96:125–133, 1954.

Scapino RP: Histopathology associated with malposition of the human temporomandibular joint disc. Oral Surg 58 375, 1984.

Stedman's Medical Dictionary, 24th ed, Baltimore, Williams & Wilkins, 1982.

Strauss F, Christen A, Weber W: The architecture of the disk of the human temporomandibular joint. Helv Odontol Acta 4:1–4, 1960.

Toller, PA: Opaque arthrography of the temporomandibular joint. Int J Oral Surg 3:17, 1974.

Warwick R, Williams PL, *Gray's Anatomy*, 36th ed. London, Churchill Livingstone, 1980, pp. 440–443.

SUGGESTED READINGS

Batson OV: The anatomist looks at the temporomandibular joint. Trans Am Acad Opthalmol Otolarygol 60:413–420, 1956.

Blaustein DI, Scapino RP: Remodeling of the temporomandibular joint disk and posterior attachment in disk displacement specimens in relation to glycosaminoglycan content. Pl Reconst Surg 78:756–764, 1986.

Boyer CC, Williams TW, Steven FH: Blood supply of the temporomandibular joint. J Dent Res 43:224, 1964.

Dubrul EL: The craniomandibular articulation. In *Sicher's Oral Anatomy* 7th ed, Chapter 4. St Louis, CV Mosby Co., 1980.

Clemente, CD: *Gray's Anatomy of the Human Body*, 30th ed. Philadelphia, Lea & Febiger, 1985, pp 338–341.

Helms C, Katzberg RW, Dolwick MF: *TMJ Internal Derangements of the Temporomandibular Joint.* San Francisco, Radiology and Research Education Foundation, 1983, pp. 1–14.

Sicher H: Functional anatomy of the temporomandibular joint. In *The Temporomandibular Joint*, Sarnat BG (Ed), Chap. 2, Springfield, Charles C Thomas, 1951.

Thilander B: Innervation of the temporomandibular disc in man. Acta Odontol Scand 22:151, 1964.

PATHOLOGIC ANATOMY OF INTERNAL DERANGEMENTS

2

The temporomandibular joint is subject to the same dysfunctions and disease processes as other synovial joints. It is convenient to divide these problems into two major categories: those that involve the articular apparatus and those that affect the joint's supporting or surrounding structures. The pathogenesis of internal derangements likely represents a sequential degeneration of structures in both categories. This chapter discusses only the pathologic anatomy of internal derangements.

The majority of patients seeking treatment for craniomandibular dysfunctions have symptoms of neuromuscular origin. The discussion of pathology in this chapter is limited to the articular disorder; discussion of the neuromuscular component of the disease process is beyond the scope of this text.

DISTURBANCES IN DISC RELATIONSHIPS

The normal position of the disc and its relationship to the condylar head and glenoid fossa/posterior slope of the eminence have been described qualitatively through localization of the posterior band (Katzberg, 1984), or quantitatively/qualitatively through identification of the position of the thin (intermediate) zone (Heffez et al., 1987). Chronic disc displacement leads to altered disc morphology that in turn interferes with interpretation of disc position (Heffez, Jordon, 1988). The anterior band may undergo resorption or folding over the intermediate zone, the posterior band becomes flattened superiorly and enlarged inferiorly, and the thin zone (presum-

ably the intermediate zone) displaces anteriorly (Figs. 2-1 and 2-2).

The displaced disc is usually described as being anteriorly (and medially) located (Figs. 2-3 and 2-4) These displacements vary in degree and present different objective signs to the clinician. As a result of this new disc position, the retrodiscal tissue is progressively pulled forward over the condylar head. The disc displacement may occur acutely or gradually. With the displacement there is simultaneous disc, retrodiscal tissue, and bone remodeling. The latter may account for the lack, in most cases, of sudden changes in the occlusion.

When the posterior band of the anteriorly displaced disc lies in any position anterior to its normal orientation, the normally loaded posterior band is also moved anteriorly, with consequent gradual transfer of loading from this rather specialized tissue to the tissue now located between the glenoid fossa and condylar head (Fig. 2–5).

As the posterior band moves anteriorly to lie between the anterior slope of the condylar head and the posterior slope of the articular eminence, this structure becomes flattened and elongated in the superior joint space. In addition, a bulge develops in the inferior joint space (Figs. 2-6 to 2-9). Internally, the fiber architecture of the disc is disrupted and a new set of transverse fibers is added (Scapino, 1984).

Heffez and Jordan (1988) developed a classification scheme for disc morphology based on examination of a series of lateral cephalometric arthrotomograms and parasagittal histologic sections. Their study described five disc shapes: normal or bow-tie shape (Fig. 1-2), straight (Fig. 2-10), bulge (Fig. 2-11), funnel (Fig. 2-

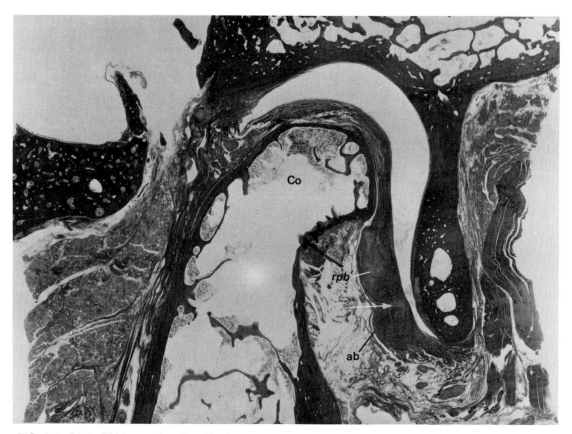

FIG. 2-1. Right TMJ; anterior disc displacement, sagittal microscopic section. The remodeled posterior band (*rpb'*) lies far anterior to the normal 1:00 o'clock position. As a result, the retrodiscal tissue has been pulled forward and overlies the anterior slope of the condylar head (Co). Closer examination would reveal extreme remodeling changes in this tissue. Note the flattening of the superior surface of the posterior band and its enlargement inferiorly. The anterior band (ab) is folded in an inferior direction, and there is an ingrowth of connective tissue in the intermediate zone (arrow)

12), and "Y" (Fig. 2-13). Certain of these alterations in disc morphology may be identified during open arthrotomies of the TMJ.

REMODELED RETRODISCAL TISSUE

The forward displacement of the disc proper can occur only in conjunction with repositioning of the retrodiscal tissue (Fig. 2-14). The disease process typi-cally appears more severe laterally, because anterior displacement usually occurs concurrently with medial displacement. Increasingly advanced stages of remodeling are usually noted from a medial to lateral direction. This was confirmed by Hansson and Oberg (1976), who examined macroscopically 115 right human temporomandibular joints and found deviations in form and arthrotic lesions located predominantly in the lateral third of the joint. Chapter 6 underscores the importance of recognizing this gradation of remodeling changes arthroscopically.

FIG. 2-3. Left TMJ; sagittal view of fresh cadaver dissection. Note, first, the anterior position of the remodeled posterior band (*rpb'*). It is positioned anterior to the eminence (E) and overlies the anterior slope of the condyle (Co). The remodeled retrodiscal tissue (*rdt'*) occupies a position between the eminence and the condylar head and is presumably undergoing pathologic loading. The flexure (fx) is formed by the junction of the remodeled retrodiscal tissue and the normal retrodiscal tissue (rdt). The glenoid fossa (GF), inferior joint space (IJS), and superior joint space (SJS) are labeled for orientation.

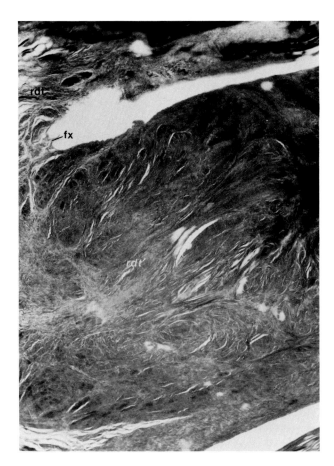

FIG. 2-2. The flexure (fx) of a chronically displaced disc. In the displaced disc, the flexure marks the junction of the tympanic portion of the retrodiscal tissue (rdt) and the remodeled retrodiscal tissue (*rdt'*). Extreme remodeling changes in the retrodiscal tissue have resulted in a dense fibrous connective tissue structure with no apparent vascularity.

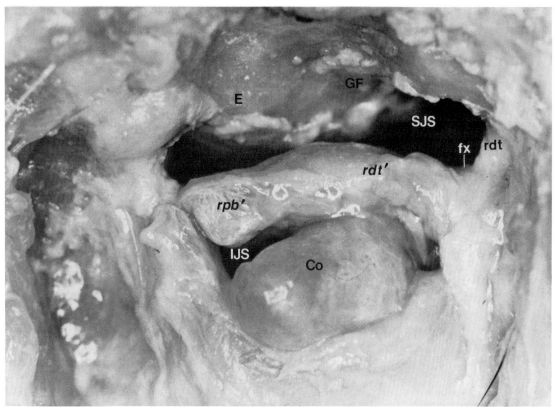

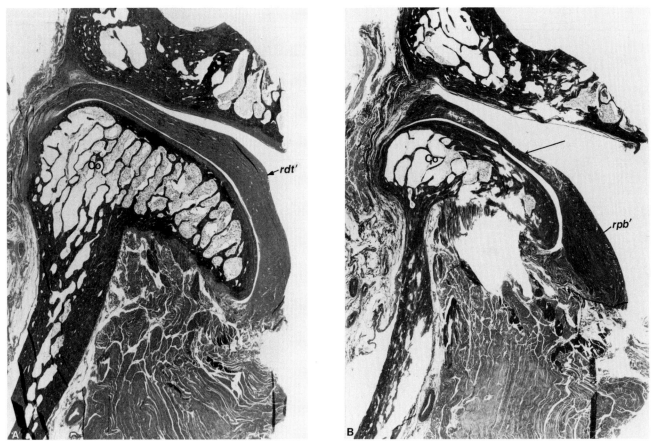

FIG. 2-4. *A*, Right TMJ; anterior (and medial) disc displacement, coronal microscopic section. Note the major remodeling changes in this remodeled retrodiscal tissue (*rdt'*) as a consequence of the anterior repositioning of this tissue over the condylar head (Co). *B*, Right temporomandibular joint; coronal microscopic section, anterior (and medial) disc displacement. This section represents a position farther anterior than that shown in Figure 2-4A. Note the extreme medial positioning of the remodeled posterior band (*rpb'*) medial to the medial pole of the condyle (Co). The remodeled retrodiscal tissue (arrow) is indicated.

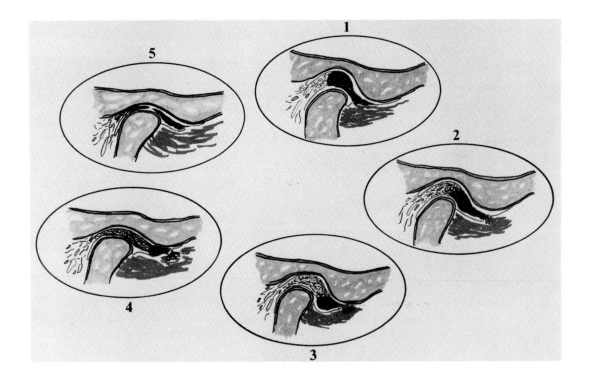

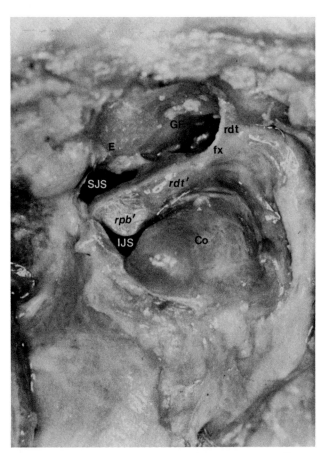

FIG. 2-6. Left TMJ; sagittal view of fresh cadaver dissection. The remodeled posterior band (*rpb'*) lies anterior to the eminence (E). The posterior band presents a pathologic morphology with its flattened superior surface and bulging inferior curvature. Remodeled retrodiscal tissue (*rdt'*) is visible overlying the condylar head (Co). Stretching of this tissue has caused the flexure (fx) to appear more U-shaped than V-shaped. Retrodiscal tissue (rdt) is seen extending posterosuperiorly from the flexure to its temporal attachment. The glenoid fossa (GF), inferior joint space (IJS), and superior joint space (SJS) are labeled for orientation.

The *flexure* in the anterior disc displacement is defined as the junction of tympanic portion of the retrodiscal tissue with the remodeled retrodiscal tissue lying over the condylar surface. The normally vascular, innervated retrodiscal tissue has an internal fiber organization that may be ill-suited to loading.

Under the functional loading of the masticatory cycle, this tissue will remodel. Functional adaptations include increasing deposition of collagen (fibrosis), increased concentrations of glycosaminoglycans (GAGs) particularly chondroitin sulfate, decreasing vascularity, and decreased innervation (Blaustein, Scapino, 1986). Probably these changes are the body's attempt to maintain a band of tissue between the condyle and the fossa. Blaustein and Scapino (1986) indicated that the posterior attachment's capacity to remodel with time changes, as not all of their specimens showed an increase in GAGs. Eventually this ill-adapted tissue becomes very thin. This process may well explain the fact that perforations of the "disc" usually occur in the retrodiscal tissue located in the position formerly occupied by the fibrous intra-articular disc. Although further investigation is necessary, these findings are consistent with the widely held theory that an anteriorly displaced disc with reduction may become nonreducing and may lead to an anteriorly displaced disc perforation. It is not clear that every individual patient goes through all of the steps of this process. Moreover, it is quite possible for a patient to pass through any of these stages so rapidly that one or another of them is clinically unobservable.

PATHOLOGY OF THE ARTICULAR SURFACES

Degenerative joint disease is known variably as *osteoarthrosis* or *osteoarthritis*. (Carlsson et al., 1979) While it is generally recognized to be a pathologic entity, its distinction from the normal remodeling processes that accompany age is not clear.

In the normally functioning joint, some subtle, adaptive changes occur constantly throughout life. The changes are the result of the joint's functional adaptations to the minor modifications of the disc-fossa relationship, tooth loss (Oberg et al., 1971), or maxillary and mandibular relationships. The most marked change found in the *normal* disc over time is the presence of chondroblasts, chondrocytes, and some hyalinization of the normally fibrous connective tissue (Moffett et al., 1964, Bhaskar, 1976). These

---

FIG. 2-5. Drawing illustrating what is believed to be the natural history of internal derangements (anterior disc displacement). *1*, Normal disc-condyle-fossa relationship; *2*, Slight anterior disc displacement; *3*, Extreme anterior disc displacement with early signs of remodeling, such as loading of retrodiscal tissue, folding/resorption of the anterior band; *4*, Long-standing anterior disc displacement with major remodeling changes in both the disc and the retrodiscal tissues; *5*, Perforation of the remodeled retrodiscal tissue establishing a pathologic communication between the superior and inferior joint spaces.

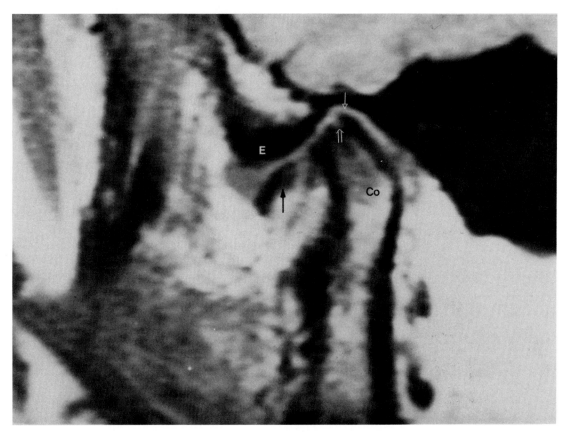

FIG. 2-7. Left TMJ in closed position; anterior disc displacement, magnetic resonance para-sagittal image (TR = 800 m sec, TE = 20 msec). The low signal intensity of the remodeled posterior band (arrow) is noted anterior to the eminence (E). The remodeled retrodiscal tissue (open arrow) appears stretched thinly where it lies over the condylar head (Co). Note the interruption of the lamina dura of the condyle (double arrow) and the invagination of tissue bearing an intermediate signal intensity.

changes are probably normal with advanced aging. Pathologic changes are thought to occur initially subsequent to a reduction of GAGs in the articular surfaces (Kopp, 1976, 1978). According to Kopp, age has no major influence on the distribution or quantity of sulfated GAGs in the normal adult (greater than 40 years) human TMJ. In displaced discs, redistribution of GAGs will occur according to the tissues loaded (Kempson et al., 1970).

The difficulty in discriminating, clinically, between normal remodeling and degeneration may explain some of the ambiguity present in the literature. Blackwood (1963) suggested a high prevalence (40%) for degenerative joint disease of the TMJ in patients over

40 years of age. On the other hand, Mayne and Hatch (1969) stated that arthritis of the TMJ was rare. Cadaveric studies by Blackwood (1963) and Macalister (1954) suggest that the disease first appears in the posterosuperior aspect of the condyle. However, the bony changes identifiable in various imaging modalities indicate the irregularities to be on the anterior and superior surfaces of the condyle (cartilage is not visible on conventional radiographs).

Macrotraumatic and microtraumatic events may be responsible for pathologic degeneration of the articular cartilages. It is likely that impulse loading places greater stresses on the joint than the oscillating forces of routine jaw function (Radin et al., 1972). Most of

FIG. 2-9. Right TMJ; anterior disc displacement, sagittal microscopic section. The posterior band exhibits remodeling changes (*rpb'*) and bulges inferiorly into the inferior joint space. The intermediate zone (iz) is seen to be anterior to its normal position where it abuts the posterior slope of the eminence (E).

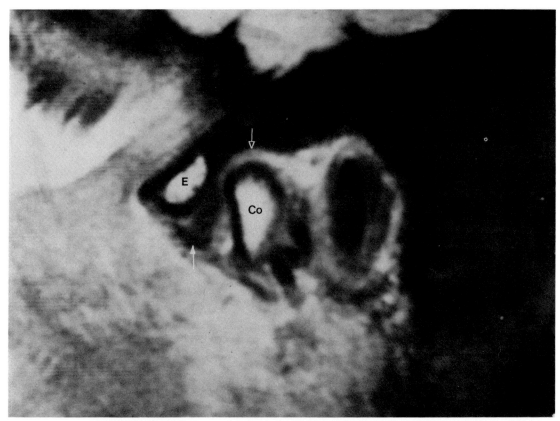

FIG. 2-8. Left TMJ in closed position; anterior disc displacement, magnetic resonance parasagittal image (TR = 800 m sec, TE = 20 msec). The remodeled posterior band (arrow) is located anterior to the eminence (E). Note its low signal intensity anterior to the condyle. The remodeled retrodiscal tissue (open arrow) is seen as a thin band of intermediate signal intensity extending from the top of the condyle (Co) anteroinferiorly over its anterior slope.

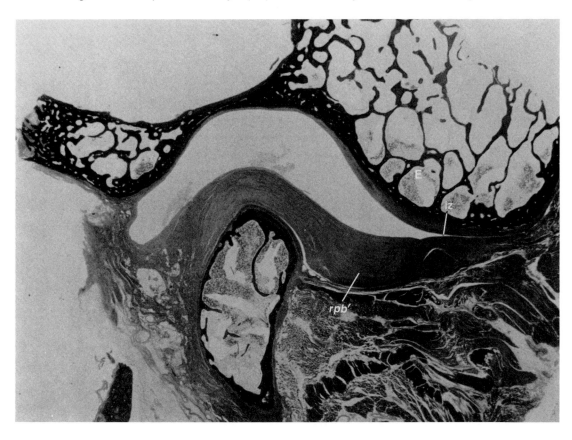

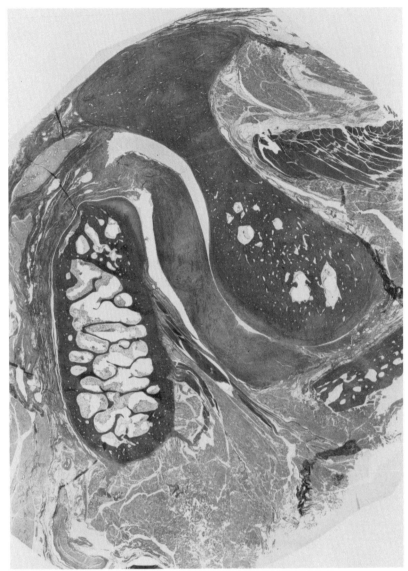

FIG. 2-10. Right TMJ; anterior disc displacement, sagittal microscopic section. Disc shape #2—straight.

the force across a joint is the product of muscle contraction rather than weight-bearing. The earliest gross finding in osteoarthosis is fibrillation of the cartilaginous surfaces, as evidenced by a change in their surface characteristics, from glossy to matte (Freeman, 1972). The degradation of cartilage proteoglycans and GAGs that leads to fibrillation does not irrevocably lead to osteoarthrosis (Maroudas et al., 1973). With cell death, lysosomes further degrade proteoglycans, resulting in decreased hard-tissue resistance to compressive forces (Ali, Evans, 1973, Kempson et al., 1970). Depletion of GAGs renders surfaces softer and more susceptible to deformation. The underlying compact bony layer then undergoes

functional remodeling, which results in stiffness. The stiffer bone is less effective as a shock absorber, and fatigue microfractures occur (Radin et al., 1972, Freeman, Kempson, 1973, Pugh et al., 1974). Subsequent denudation of the articular surface with release of necrotic cartilage tissue can cause a synovitis with eventual fibrosis and capsular contraction. Osseous remodeling may lead to osteolysis of the subchondral cancellous bone, further reducing its resistance to mechanical loading (Bean et al., 1977, Lereim et al., 1974). According to Oberg et al., 1971), the greatest remodeling changes occur on the lateroposterior aspect of the eminence and anterior portion of the condyle. Hypervascular areas surrounding load areas

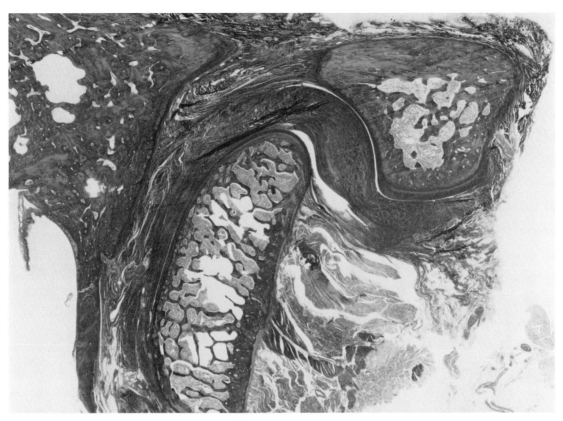

FIG. 2-11. Right TMJ; anterior disc displacement, sagittal microscopic section. Disc shape #3—bulge.

FIG. 2-12. Right TMJ; anterior disc displacement, sagittal microscopic section. Disc shape #4—funnel.

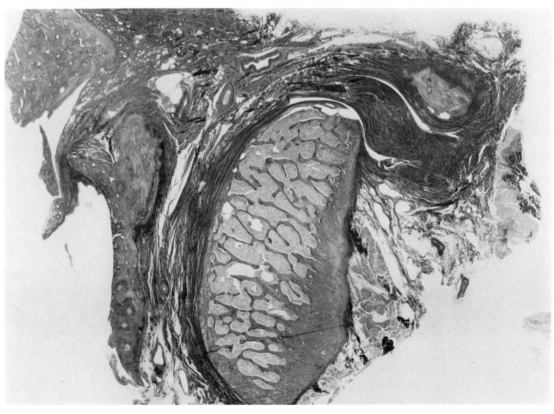

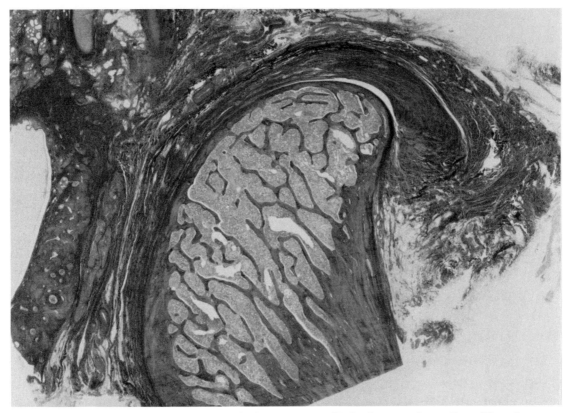

FIG. 2-13. Right TMJ; anterior disc displacement, sagittal microscopic section. Disc shape #5—Y.

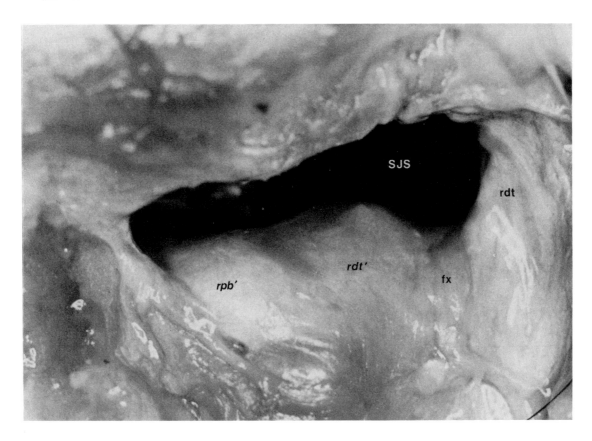

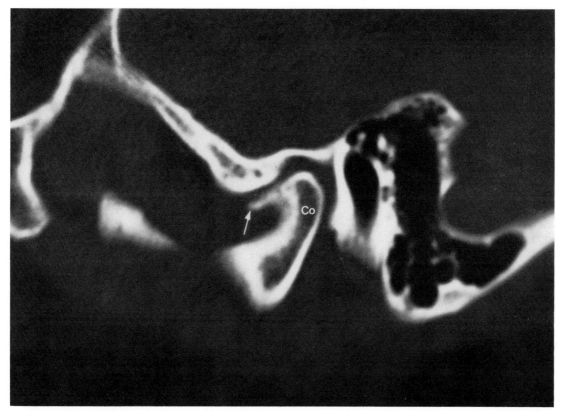

FIG. 2-15. CT scan of left TMJ. A long, thin, sharply pointed osteophyte (arrow) is seen extending anteriorly from the condylar head (Co).

may show new bone formations called *osteophytes* (Jeffrey, 1973).

Sclerosis of the condylar lamina dura, the radiologic sign of subchondral trabecular stiffening and one of the earliest radiographic signs seen, is not always noted (Toller, 1973). Most consistent radiographic signs include either a loss of density or an interruption in the lamina dura of the condyle. The loss of density may represent the subarticular false cysts described in other osteoarthrotic joints (Landells, 1953). A scooped-out erosion in the cortical bone with a sharp periphery is a typical finding in more advanced disease. The bony irregularities may be of sufficient magnitude to demonstrate radiologic evidence of osteophyte formation (Fig. 2-15).

Whether disc displacement is a prerequisite for osseous and cartilaginous degeneration or remodeling is not clear. According to Toller (1973), clicking is usually absent, and crepitus is frequent in the osteoarthrotic joint. Concomitant chronic disc and retrodiscal tissue remodeling changes may account for this clinical finding. Radiographically, evidence of degenerative changes seems to be particularly prominent in TMJs with retrodiscal tissue perforations (Figs. 2-7 and 2-8).

Chapters 5 and 6 will show that arthroscopy offers the clinician an opportunity to readily examine the condition of the glenoid fossa/eminence articular surfaces. Surface irregularities of the condylar head may be visible during examination of the superior joint

FIG. 2-14. Left TMJ; sagittal view, fresh cadaver dissection with an anteriorly displaced disc seen from above. The convexity of the remodeled retrodiscal tissue (*rdt'*) results from the position of the condylar head beneath it. In a normal disc-condyle-fossa relationship, the condylar head would underly the posterior band. Note the remodeled posterior band (*rpb'*). The flexure (fx) is seen at the junction of the remodeled retrodiscal tissue and the *normal* retrodiscal tissue (rdt). The superior joint space (SJS) is labeled for orientation. The inferior joint space is not exposed.

space when retrodiscal tissue perforations are present (Plate 41). In the future, arthroscopy may help to resolve some of the lingering questions about the pathogenesis of internal derangements and osteoarthrosis.

REFERENCES

Ali SY, Evans I: Enzymatic degradation of cartilage in osteoarthrosis. Fed Proc **32**:1494, 1973.

Bhasker SN (ed): Orban's oral histology and Embryology. St. Louis, CV Mosby Co, 1976, pp 395–404.

Blackwood HJ Jr: Arthritis of the mandibular joint. Br Dent J *115*:317–326, 1963.

Blaustein DI, Scapino RP: Remodeling of the temporomandibular joint disk and posterior attachment in disk displacement specimens in relation to glycosaminoglycan content. Pl Reconst Surg *78*:756–764, 1986.

Carlsson GE, Kopp S, Oberg T, In: Zarb GA, Carlsson GE (ed). *Temporomandibular Joint Function and Dysfunction*. Copenhagen, Munksgaard, 1979, pp. 269–293.

Freeman MAR: The pathogenesis of osteoarthrosis: an hypothesis. In: Appley, AG (ed.). *Modern Trends in Orthopaedics*. London Butterworhs, Vol. 6, 1972, p. 40.

Freeman MAR, Kempson GE: Load carriage. In: Freeman MAR (ed) *Adult Articular Cartilage*. Oxford Pitman Medical, Alden Press, 1973, pp. 228–246.

Hansson T, Oberg T: Arthrosis and deviation in form in the temporomandibular joint. A macroscopic study on a human autopsy material. Acta Odont Scand 35:167–174, 1976.

Heffez L, Jordan S: A classification of TMJ disc morphology. Oral Surg, Oral Med, Oral Path 67:11–19, 1989.

Heffez L, Jordan S, Going R: Determination of the radiographic position of the temporomandibular joint disc. Oral Surg, Oral Med, Oral Path 65:272–280, 1988.

Jeffrey AK: Osteogenesis in the osteoarthritic femoral head. A study using radioactive ^{32}P and tetracycline bone markers. J Bone Joint Surg(Br) 55:262–272, 1973.

Katzberg RW. Third Annual meeting temporomandibular joint pain and dysfunction. Nov 2–4, 1984, Philadelphia, Pennsylvania

Kempson GE, Muir H, Swanson SAV et al. Correlations between stiffness and chemical constituents of cartilage on the human femoral head. Biochem Biophys Acta *215*:70, 1970.

Kopp S: Topographical distribution of sulfated glycosaminoglycans in human temporomandibular joint disks. A histochemical study of autopsy material. J Oral Path 5:265–276, 1976.

Kopp S: Topographical distribution of sulfated glycosaminoglycans in the surface layers of the human temporomandibular joint. J Oral Path 7:283–294, 1978.

Landells JW: The bone cysts of osteoarthritis. J Bone J Surg(Br), *35B*:643–649, 1953.

Lereim P, Goldie I, Dahlberg E: Hardness of the subchondral bone of the tibial condyles in the normal state and in osteoarthritis and rheumatoid arthritis. Acta Orthop Scand 45:614, 1974.

Macalister AD:A microscopic survey of the human temporomandibular joint. N Z Dent J, *50*:161, 1954.

Maroudas A, Evans H, Almeida L: Cartilage of the hip joint: topographical variation of glycosaminoglycan content in normal and fibrillated tissue. Ann Rheum Dis *32*(1): 1973.

Mayne JG, Hatch GS: Arthritis of the temporomandibular joint. JADA *79*:125-130, 1969.

Moffett BC, Johnson LC, McCabe JB, et al. Articular remodeling in the adult human temporomandibular joint. Am J Anat 115:119–141, 1964.

Oberg T, Carlsson GE, Fajers CM: The temporomandibular joint. A morphologic study on a human autopsy material. Acta Odont Scand 29:349–384, 1971.

Pugh JW, Radin EL, Rose RM: Quantitative studies of human subchondral cancellous bone: its relationship to the state of its overlying cartilage. J Bone Joint Surg (Am) 56:313–321, 1974.

Radin El, Paul IL, Rose RM: Role of mechanical factors in pathogenesis of primary osteoarthritis. Lancet, 1:519–521, 1972.

Scapino RP: Histopathology associated with malposition of the human temporomandibular joint disc. Oral Surg 58:375, 1984.

Toller PA: Osteoarthrosis of the mandibular condyle. Brit Dent J *134*:223–231, 1973.

SUGGESTED READINGS

Bean LR, Omnell K-A, Oberg T: Comparison between radiologic observations and macroscopic tissue changes in temporomandibular joints. Dentomaxillofac Radiol 6:90, 1977.

Hall MB, Brown RW & Baughman RA: Histologic appearance of the bilaminar zone in internal derangement of the temporomandibular joint. Oral Surg 58:375–381, 1984.

Helms C, Katzberg RW, Dolwick MF: *TMJ Internal Derangements of the Temporomandibular Joint*. San Francisco, Radiology and Research Education Foundation, 1983, pp. 1–14

Isberg A, Isaacsson G: Tissue reactions of the temporomandibular joint following retrusive guidance of the mandible. J Craniomand Prac 4:143, 1986.

Oberg T, Carlsson GE: Macroscopic and microscopic anatomy of the temporomandibular joint. In: Zarb GA, Carlsson GE (ed). *Temporomandibular Joint Function and Dysfunction*. Copenhagen, Munksgaard, 1979, pp. 15–63.

ARTHROSCOPIC INSTRUMENTATION, STERILIZATION, AND PHOTOGRAPHY

3

INSTRUMENTATION

THE ARTHROSCOPE

This discussion of arthroscopic instrumentation is divided into three sections. The first section discusses the arthroscope proper. The second section discusses the solid instruments for penetration of the joint space and for manipulation of intra-articular structures. The third section discusses the equipment required to provide adequate illumination.

The arthroscope is essentially a cylinder that conducts light into a cavity and transmits an image back to the eye. The telescope is made of several components common to all endoscopic systems. They include an ocular lens mounted on an eyepiece; an illuminating mechanism; a transmitting mechanism consisting of a series of lenses or a fiber(s); and a working end consisting of a prism and an objective (Fig. 3-1).

Several small-joint arthroscopic systems are currently available for examining the temporomandibular joint. The optical principles of each telescopic system fall into one of three categories: traditional lens system, selfoscope lens system, and rod lens system. The traditional lens system and the rod lens system are examples of *rigid endoscopy*, in which the transmitting mechanism is a series of lenses and the illuminating mechanism is a fiber bundle. The selfoscope system is somewhere between rigid endoscopy and *fiberoptic endoscopy*. Although it uses glass fibers in both its transmitting and illuminating mechanisms, it does not fulfill the criteria of flexibility that

would make it an example of fiberoptic endoscopy (Fig. 3-2). In fiberoptic endoscopy, the specific arrangement of the transmitting fibers at the working end is continued to the eyepiece (coherence of fiber bundles) to prevent scrambling and distortion of the image. This coherent fiber arrangement is much more complex than the incoherent fiber bundle arrangement of the rigid endoscope's fiber light cable.

Traditional Lens System (Fig. 3-3)

The traditional optical system consists of a long, narrow tube with a series of small glass relay and field lenses assembled at specific intervals with intervening air spaces. To reduce the effect of stray light on the contrast of the final image, the inner surface of the tube is corrugated or "rifled" (Fig. 3-4).

Selfoscope Lens System (Fig. 3-5)

The selfoscope system consists of a long, narrow tube containing a single image-transmitting fiber and multiple incoherent illuminating fibers. The transmitting fiber, diameter 0.5 to 1.0 mm, is specially treated to improve its refractive index.

The engineering of the selfoscope system allows fabrication of systems with an external diameter as small as 1.7 mm. However, limitations in the degree of brightness, viewing angle, color, resolution, and contrast of the selfoscope system makes it less desirable, in our opinion, than the rod lens system (Fig. 3-6).

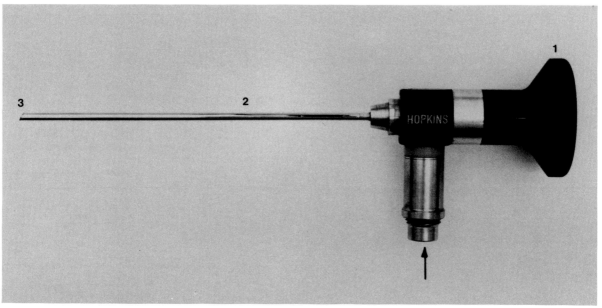

FIG. 3-1. 1, The arthroscope eyepiece. 2, illuminating and transmitting mechanisms housed within the rigid cylinder. 3, objective. The illumination source is coupled to the inlet post (arrow).

Rod Lens System (Fig. 3-7)

The rod lens optical system reverses the function of air and glass from that used in the traditional system. Air lenses (rather than glass) and glass spaces are used to improve light transmission. The capacity of the telescope to transmit light is directly proportional to the square of the refractive index of the relay lenses. The glass spaces of the rod lens system have an index of approximately 1.50 to 1.60. This index compares favorably to that of air (n = 1.00).

The rod lens system has several advantages over the other systems (Figs. 3-4 and 3-5). A brighter image results from decreased light absorption. The diagnostic capability is improved owing to the wider viewing angle. The key to arthroscopy is gaining orientation by establishing topographic relationships. The rod lens system provides improved contrast, color reproduction, and resolution. These advantages have facilitated the development of auxiliary instruments for diagnostic and surgical arthroscopy. The arthro-

FIG. 3-2. The fiberscope. Note that a coherent fiber bundle serves as the transmitting mechanism. Compare with Fig. 3-6, in which the transmitting mechanism is a series of relay and field lenses. (Reprinted with permission from Berci G: Endoscopy. New York, Appleton-Century-Crofts, 1976.)

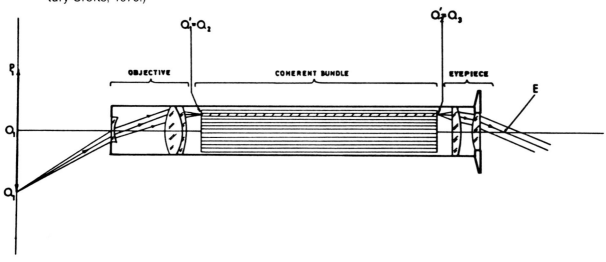

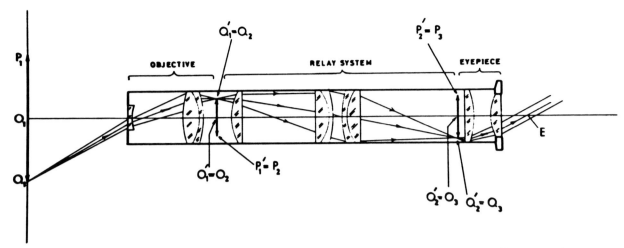

FIG. 3-3. Traditional endoscope. Image formation depends on a combination of lenses at the distal end of the telescope to form a reduced image (the objective), several unit-magnification relay systems to refocus the light (the relay and field lenses), and a combination of lenses at the proximal end to produce a magnified, virtual image of the final relayed image (the eyepiece). (Reprinted with permission from Berci G: Endoscopy. New York, Appleton-Century-Crofts, 1976.)

FIG. 3-4. The assembly of the traditional endoscope (*A*) and the rod lens telescope (*B*). Note the *rifling* of the inner aspect of the traditional endoscope's tube to suppress incident light, which would severely degrade the contrast of the transmitted image. Rifling decreases the inner aperture radius ρ_1 and thus light transmission. (Reprinted with permission from Berci G: Endoscopy. New York, Appleton-Century-Crofts, 1976.)

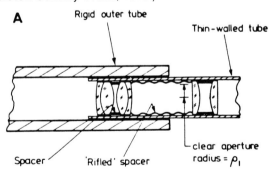

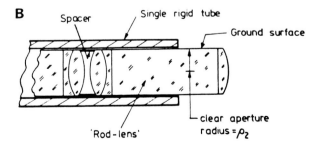

scopic illustrations chosen for this text were obtained with the 2.4-mm Karl Storz rod lens telescope. To date, the complexity of assembling the 30 degree forward-oblique rod lens telescope system has limited its minimum external diameter to 1.9 mm. The diameter of this instrument does not pose a problem in accessing the superior joint space; however, with industry competition, smaller-diameter forward-oblique viewing rod lens telescopes will surely be developed. Whether these telescopes will adversely limit the field of view and restrict diagnostic and operative capabilities is as yet unknown (Fig. 3-7).

Available telescopes vary in their *direction of view.* The objective lens may be mounted at 0, 10, 25, 30, 70, or 120 degrees (Fig. 3-8). The most versatile telescope and the one preferred by most arthroscopists has a direction of view between 25 and 30 degrees. This telescope may be rotated in place to increase the *field of view (vision)* to approximately 75 degrees (Fig. 3-9). *Field of view* is defined as the conical area determined by the outer limits at which portions of an object or objects are perceived. When a pediatric urethrotome is used for surgery, a telescope with a 0 degree direction of view is employed to permit simultaneous visualization of the cutting instrument and those tissues targeted by the cutting instrument (Fig. 3-10). This instrument may be adopted for temporomandibular joint arthroscopic surgery (Fig. 3-11). Increasing the direction of view to 70 degrees increases the field of view but creates a large blind spot directly in front of it. This field of view obtains an

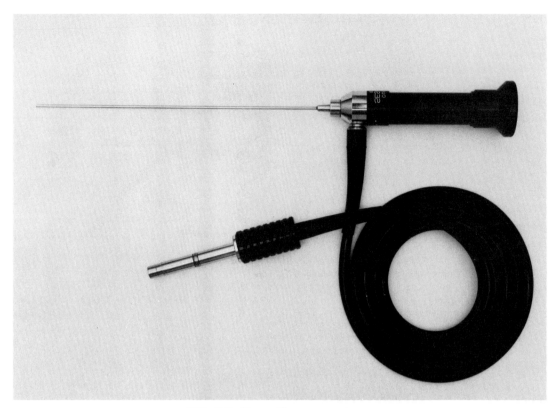

FIG. 3-5. The selfoscope system.

FIG. 3-6. A photograph obtained with the selfoscope lens system. Compare with plates in Chapters 5 to 7.

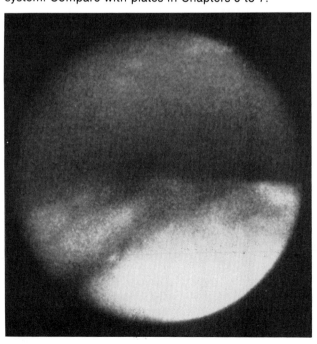

excellent side view (Fig. 3-12). Direction of view and field of view should not be confused. Figure 3-13 illustrates these concepts (Berci 1975, Shahriaree, 1984, Heffez, Blaustein 1987).

SOLID INSTRUMENTS

The basic instruments for penetration and exploration of the joint are the same for each arthroscopic system. These instruments are categorized as *capsule penetration* instruments, *hand-held* surgical instruments, and *motorized* surgical instruments.

Capsule Penetration Instruments

For capsule penetration, each system contains three principal components: external sheath, sharp trocar (obturator), and blunt trocar (Fig. 3-14). Small differences in design exist, such as the length of instruments and the type of locking mechanisms (spring versus manual). The choice of one instrument design over another is largely governed by operator preference.

External sheaths, blunt trocars, and sharp trocars of varying diameters and lengths are available to ac-

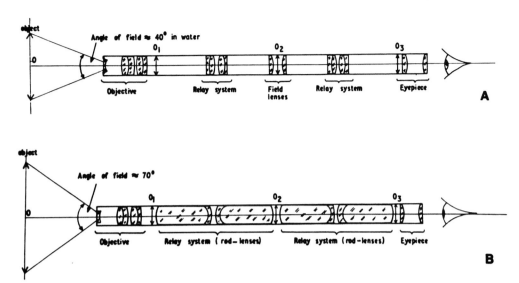

FIG. 3-7. The optics of a traditional endoscope (*A*) and the rod lens system (*B*). The traditional lens system is composed of a series of glass field and relay lenses and air spaces. The rod lens system is composed of air lenses and glass spaces. For the same number of relay stages, the rod lens increases its light-transmitting capacity twofold, because of the refractive index of the glass spaces. (Reprinted with permission from Berci G: Endoscopy. New York, Appleton-Century-Crofts, 1976.)

FIG. 3-8. Three telescopes with varying directions of view are illustrated. If the optical axis (OA) of the telescope is extrapolated, the deviation from the horizontal optical axis measures the direction of view (DV). *1*, Straightforward view (0 degree). *2*, Forward-oblique view (30 degree). *3*, Forward-oblique view (70 degree).

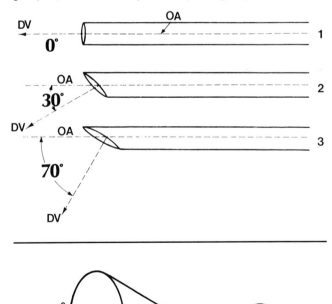

FIG. 3-9. Rotating a 30 degrees forward-oblique viewing telescope about its axis increases its field of view to 75 degrees. The increase in field of view is depicted by the dotted circle. In the lower left corner, the fields of view of a 0 degree (solid circle) viewing telescope and a 30 degree (dotted circle) viewing telescope rotated about their axes are composed. (Adapted with permission from Shahriaree H: O'Connor's Textbook of Arthroscopic Surgery, Philadelphia, JB Lippincott Co., 1984.)

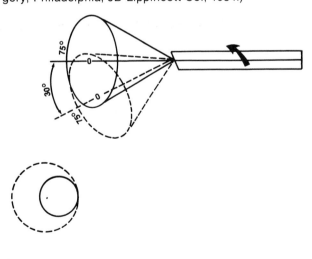

FIG. 3-10. The field of view of the straightforward viewing telescope is depicted. In the lower left corner, one can see that rotating the telescope about its axis does not increase the field of view. (Adapted with permission from Shahriaree H: O'Connor's Textbook of Arthroscopic Surgery, Philadelphia, JB Lippincott Co., 1984.)

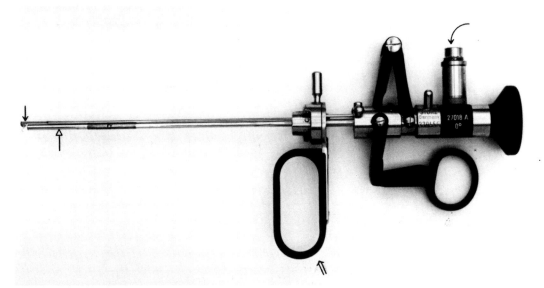

FIG. 3-11. A pediatric urethrotome (resectoscope) may be adapted for operative arthroscopy. A 0 degree viewing telescope (open arrow) is mounted in conjunction with a cutting instrument (arrow). Depressing the trigger control (double arrow) allows the cutting instrument to leave the protective external sheath, not shown here (see Fig. 3-17). Curved arrow indicates the post for coupling of the fiber light cable to the telescope.

comodate hand and motor instruments or to act as an outflow port when a two-port system is used (Fig. 3-15).

Hand-Held Instruments

A probe (Fig. 3-16A,B) is an effective tool in both diagnostic and operative arthroscopy. By virtue of the

FIG. 3-12. Rotating a 70 degree forward-oblique viewing telescope about its axis increases its field of view. Note the large blind spot created directly in front of the telescope. The increase in field of view and central blind spot are shown in the lower left corner. (Adapted with permission from Shahriaree H: O'Connor's Textbook of Arthroscopic Surgery. Philadelphia, JB Lippincott Co., 1984.)

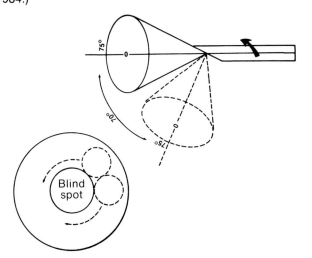

FIG. 3-13. Viewing angle (VA) is shown with dotted lines. The 60 degrees viewing angle is formed by the two outer visual limits. The direction of view (DV) corresponds to the bisector of the viewing angle. Various directions of view with a 60 degree viewing angle are illustrated. (Optical axis, OA) (Reprinted with permission from Endoscopy, George Berci, New York, Appleton-Century-Crofts, 1976.)

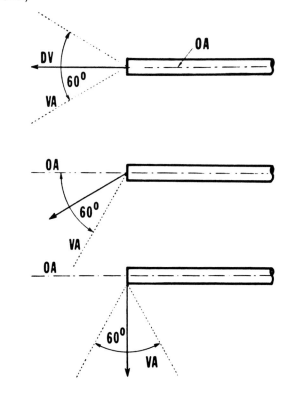

FIG. 3-14. A, 2.4 mm, 30 degree forward-oblique viewing telescope; eyepiece-objective length 23 cm. B, 2.4 mm, 30 degree forward-oblique viewing telescope; eyepiece-objective length 15.1 cm. C, 2.7-mm external sheath D, Blunt trocar. E, sharp trocar. Note the site for attachment of the light cable on the telescopes (curved arrows). Note the site on the external sheath for attachment of the extension tube for irrigation (straight arrow).

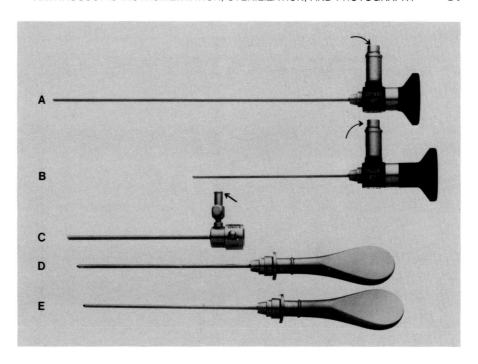

dull hook at its distal end, the probe may be used to practice triangulation, retract the retrodiscal tissue, and check the consistency of remodeled retrodiscal tissue and disc.

The pediatric urethrotome may be adapted for operative arthroscopy (Figs. 3-11 and 3-17). This instrument can be used as a single instrument for diagnostic and operative arthroscopy. A 0 degree telescope is mounted in tandem to a cutting instrument. The external sheath can thus accommodate the telescope, cutting instrument, and irrigant. Rosette, straight, sickle, and retrograde knives are available (Fig. 3-18).

A trigger allows the operator to control the movement of the knife in and out of the external sheath. The external sheath is elliptical and measures 4 millimeters in maximum diameter. This instrument may be useful in cutting diseased tissue. The arthroscopist may initially encounter several difficulties with the field of view afforded through the 0 degree telescope. In addition, the diameter of the external sheath may, in some cases, restrict mobility. With practice, however, this instrument has proven effective in cutting portions of the remodeled retrodiscal tissue.

Scissors and punch forceps with long working arms

FIG. 3-15. Trocars of various diameters (2.6, 2.8, 3.5 mm) (*A*) and appropriate sheaths (B) for establishment of the second port.

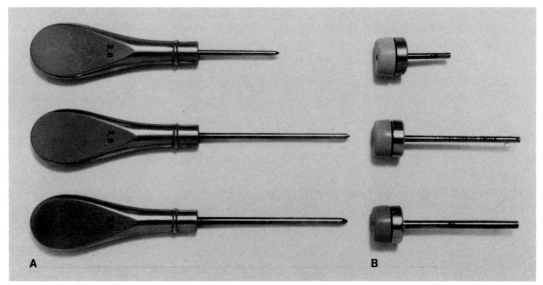

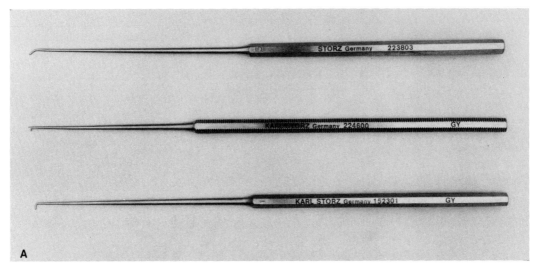

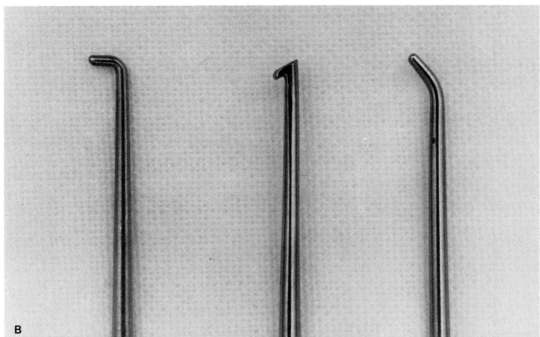

FIG. 3-16. *A*, Arthroscopic probes. *B*, Close-up of arthroscopic probes.

may be introduced through the external sheath of the second port. A variety of instrument designs permit the retrieval of foreign bodies, removal of small pieces of tissue, and incision of adhesions (Figs. 3-19 and 3-20).

A variety of arthroscopic knives (Figs. 3-21 and 3-22) with different configurations may be used to incise tissue. These instruments have proven to be most effective in cutting remodeled retrodiscal tissue. They pass readily through the short external sheath of the second port. Unfortunately, they need to be replaced frequently because they dull quickly, and the various blade configurations make resharpening difficult. The cutting edges may best be maintained by preventing contact with each other and other objects. Red rubber or silicone tubing may be used to cover the edges. However, this protection may interfere with adequate sterilization.

A malleable tension arm (Fig. 3-23) is available to assist in holding the telescope during operative arthroscopy. The arm attaches to the side of the operating table. The tension of the arm may be adjusted so that it can carry the telescope with the weight of a video camera or articulated arm.

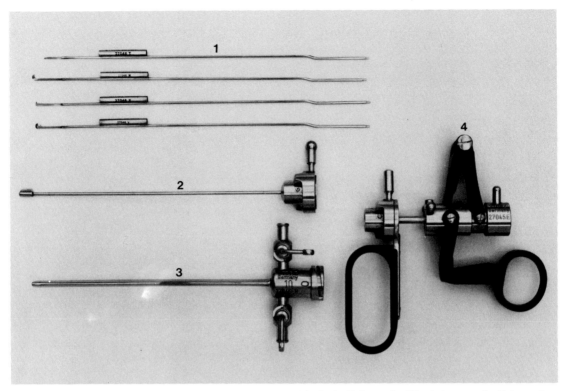

FIG. 3-17. The pediatric urethrotome disassembled. 1, Knives. 2, Blunt trocar. 3, External sheath (4 mm maximum diameter). 4, Attachment with trigger control.

FIG. 3-18. Various blade designs are available for the pediatric urethrotome. Rosette, straight, sickle, and retrograde knives are shown (left to right).

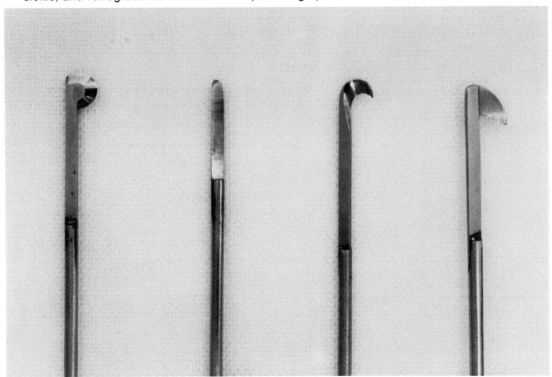

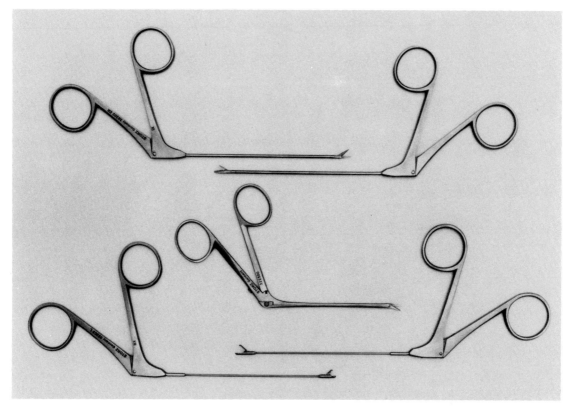

FIG. 3-19. Arthroscopic scissors.

FIG. 3-20. Close-up of microscissors demonstrating (from left to right) biopsy forceps, grasping scissors, sharp-nosed scissors, up-biting scissors, and down-biting scissors.

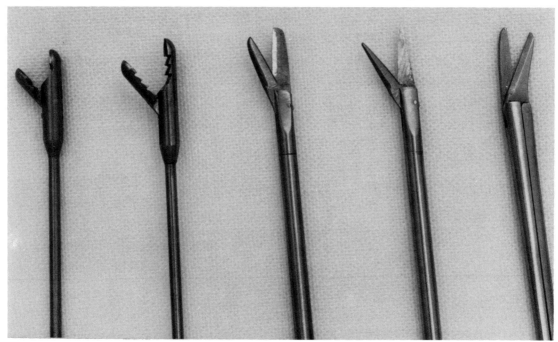

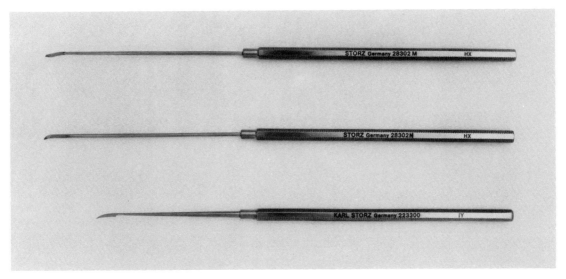

FIG. 3-21. Arthroscopic knives.

Motorized Instruments

The shaver (Fig. 3-24) consists of a hollow, distally fenestrated sheath containing a rotating cylindric cutting instrument that can rotate within the hollow sheath. A variety of cutting instruments are available (Fig. 3-25). The cutting instruments are driven by a motor, controlled by a foot pedal. Cable-driven and battery-powered models, as well as shavers containing power components, are available. Each type of shaver has its restrictions with regard to sterilization.

The efficiency of the cutting instrument depends on several factors, including the strength of the motor, the proximity of the cutting instrument to the edge of the fenestration in the outer sheath, and the diameter of the lumen of the sheath. The cutting instruments dull rapidly. The handle of the shaver has an attachment for suction that the arthroscopist may opt to apply while cutting. In this case, the debris is sucked up into the hollow sheath and immediately removed from the joint space. Although these instruments have proven their efficacy in removal of

FIG. 3-22. Close-up of three arthroscopic knives demonstrating two different blade configurations.

FIG. 3-23. One end of the malleable tension arm attaches to the side of the operating table (arrow), while the other end holds the telescope in place (open arrow).

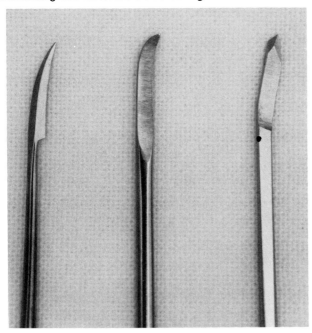

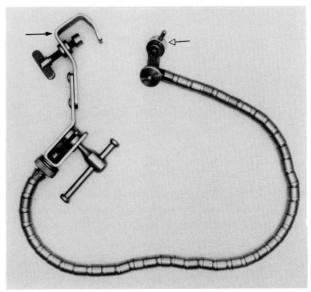

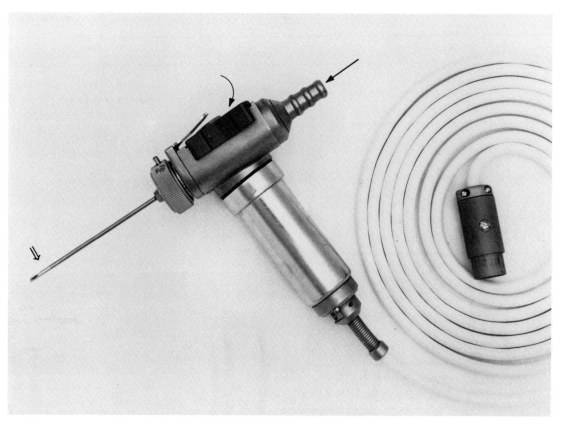

FIG. 3-24. Motorized shaver. Fenestrated aperture (double arrow), control for suction (curved arrow), and site of connection for suction tube (arrow) are indicated.

FIG. 3-25. Various cutting instruments (*A*) and fenestrated sheaths (*B*) for the motorized shaver.

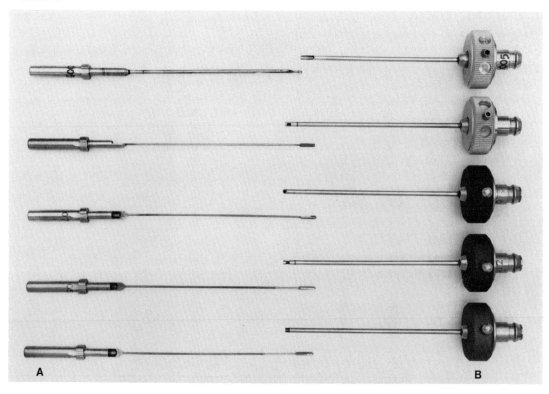

A   B

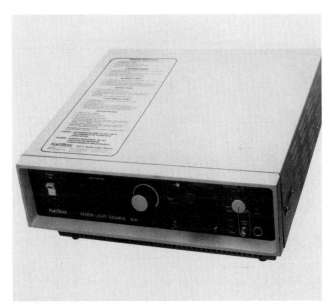

FIG. 3-26. Xenon light source, 6000 Kelvin degrees (approx), 300 watts. This light source provides the optimum illumination for still and video photography. In addition, a rapid recharge time and an audible "ready" signal facilitate photography.

fibrillated or fragmented knee articular cartilage or hypertrophied synovium, they do not effectively cut intact remodeled retrodiscal tissue. When the fenestrated portion of the sheath is applied to the tissue and the motor activated, the tissue is pinched be-

tween the blade of the cutting instrument and the aperture, and the tissue then severed. The assistant must maintain adequate distension of the joint space to prevent collapse of the joint and sucking of the retrodiscal tissue into the aperture of the instrument, which occurs when the inflow capacity is exceeded by the outflow capacity (suction) (Shahriaree, Erichsen, 1984).

ILLUMINATION

Several types of light sources are available. Xenon light (Fig. 3-26) provides brighter images with better color rendition than halogen light. Compare Plate 6, obtained with a xenon light source with Plate 3, obtained with a halogen light source. Typically, 150-watt tungsten halogen and 6000-Kelvin, 300-watt xenon sources are available. Lamp output is adjustable. A series of adapters are sold to enable light cables of one manufacturer to match the light source of another. If still photography is important to the operator, a light source that offers the option of regulating light discharge with a TTL (through the lens) cable is a significant accessory (Fig. 3-27).

Fiber light cables (Fig. 3-28) are used for illumination only. As stated earlier, they are composed of incoherent fiber bundles. Each cable contains multiple fiberglass threads that conduct light from the light source through the telescope and into the articular

FIG. 3-27. Close-up of operating panel of xenon light source (Fig. 3-26). Intensity controls are to the left, and automatic flash generator for still photography, with TTL cable attachment, to the right. The site of attachment of the fiberoptic cable is indicated (arrow).

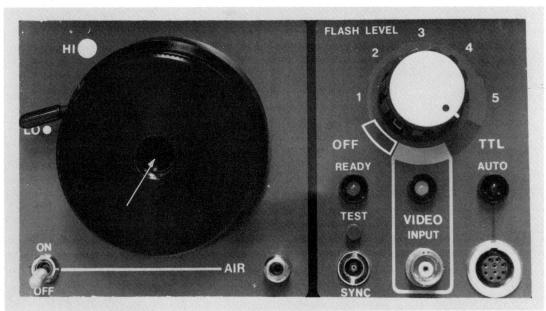

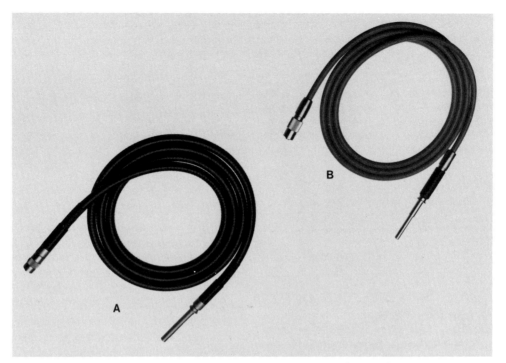

FIG. 3-28. Fluid (*A*) and fiber (*B*) light cables. The fluid cable is less flexible than the fiber cable, but is recommended where optimum color transmission is desired.

cavity. Each fiber has a diameter of about 25 μ and is composed of two types of high-quality optical glass. A high refractive index core transmits light, and a low refractive index cladding provides internal reflection for optimum conservation of light. Light may be internally reflected more than 15,000 times per meter in a fiberglass light guide. Without the cladding, contamination of the surface of the fiber would cause significant loss of light. The cable is fragile and must not be bent or coiled tightly. In general, cables should be cold sterilized. Some manufacturers permit autoclaving. The integrity of the fiber cable may be verified by turning the light source to a low intensity and checking the distal end for black voids. Fiber cables of varying lengths and diameters are available. Increasing the diameter of the fiber cable increases the amount of light conducted from the light source. However, the amount of light entering the joint cavity cannot be increased beyond the optimum light-conducting efficiency of the finite number of fibers in the telescope. Poor coupling of the fiber cable to the telescope will result in significant loss of light.

Fluid light cables (Fig. 3-28) are also available. These cables conduct light through a fluid medium. Photographic images will appear brighter. These cables are less flexible, and the operator may initially find their stiffness difficult to manage. (Berci, 1976)

STERILIZATION

The telescopes should be carefully inspected before and after every arthroscopic procedure to ensure that they have been properly handled and are free of damage and to verify the clarity of view. Ocular and objective lenses should also be checked using incidental light.

All surfaces must be properly cleaned prior to sterilization. The adaptors for the light cable should be unscrewed and the surface of the inlet cleaned with mild detergent and water (pH 7.0 to 8.5), using a cotton tip applicator. The telescopes should be cleaned in a similar manner. The ocular and objective lenses should be cleaned with 70% isopropyl alcohol and dried with compressed air or a soft, fine linen cloth (Karl Storz, 1988). Ultrasonic cleaning should be avoided as it may contribute to the loosening of soldered joints. Surface corrosion of stainless steel may be minimized by soaking instruments in a water-soluble instrument "milk" bath and lubricating their mechanical joints.

Most of the other arthroscopic equipment may be gas or steam autoclaved. Repeated steam autoclaving of the telescopes shortens their lives. A telescope is essentially a metallic tube with a series of glass parts. Rapid temperature changes associated with steam sterilization cause differential thermal expansion and contraction of glass and metallic parts. Condensation will appear on the lenses if air is able to enter the endoscope through a crack or a broken seal. Gas sterilization with ethylene oxide remains the preferred method. However, most hospitals insist on a mandatory aeration period of 12 to 24 hours with this technique. Immediately following gas sterilization, the residual ethylene oxide content falls below the 250 ppm maximum recommended level for devices contacting mucosa or skin (Fed. Reg. vol 43, No. 122, Fri. June 23, 1978, Part 5, p. 27474-27483). At least one manufacturer states that its telescopes require no aeration when they are wrapped in a special foam-lined case (Karl Storz, 1988).

If equipment is insufficient to accommodate more than one arthroscopic procedure per day, cold sterilization with 2% glutaraldehyde solution may be used for the telescopes. The telescopes must not soak for more than 20 minutes, as the seals around the objective and ocular lenses may deteriorate with repeated prolonged soakings. Johnson et al. (1982) confirmed that this method was a safe, effective means of sterilization. They reported an infection rate of 0.04% using a 15-minute soak in 2% activated glutaraldehyde. The fiberoptic light cables and video camera can only be cold sterilized, unless the manufacturer specifies otherwise. The articulated arms cannot be sterilized and must be draped with sterile sleeves (Nemethy 1976, Shahriaree, Erichsen, 1984).

PHOTOGRAPHY IN ARTHROSCOPY

The need for good documentation of arthroscopic procedures arose because of the widespread acceptance of diagnostic and surgical arthroscopy by the orthopedic community. As endoscopic surgical procedures are developed for the treatment of internal derangements of the temporomandibular joint, communication of methods and results will necessitate knowledge of endoscopic photographic techniques.

Whether the operator regards himself as primarily a diagnostic arthroscopist or a surgical arthroscopist, the photographic record is of value. The diagnostician may prefer to perform conventional surgery after the specific pathologic condition has been identified, or may on the basis of the examination decide to obtain a consultation prior to surgery. In any case, the photographic record is invaluable. An accurate photographic record provides some degree of medicolegal protection. Videotapes and slide material are excellent teaching aids and may be used in publications.

Historically, the advancement and eventual adoption of the endoscopic technique as an established orthopedic procedure was based on the development of sophisticated photographic methods.

For *still photography* the following equipment is recommended:

1. Rod lens telescope.
2. 35-mm single-lens-reflex camera adaptable to the arthroscope. (Fig. 3-29)
3. Ektachrome 400 ASA (Eastman Kodak Company, Rochester, New York) for diapositives and Kodacolor 400 ASA (Eastman Kodak Company) for prints.
4. A xenon light source, though a 150-watt halogen light source is acceptable (Figs. 3-26 and 3-27).
5. Light source capable of regulating flash discharge typically with a TTL cable connecting the camera to the light source.
6. Lens with a focal length of 60 to 130 mm. Optimal photographs have been obtained with magnification of 90 to 110 × (Fig. 3-29).
7. Tripod or stabilizing arm for the camera.
8. Optical teaching attachment with rod lens system (articulating arm) to connect the telescope to the camera. Two-, three-, and four-joint articulating arms are available (Fig. 3-30).
9. Optional accessories include a data back system and motor drive.

The following additional equipment is recommended for *video photography*:

1. Lightweight video camera. (Fig. 3-31).
2. Video recorder. Preferably, a ¾-inch videotape recorder should be employed to permit optimal image resolution. Significant resolution is lost with second and third generation edited ½-inch videotapes. With advances in the video industry, higher resolution ½-inch videotapes may soon appear on the market.

FIG. 3-29. 35-mm single-lens reflex camera with telescopic lens of focal length 60 to 130 mm.

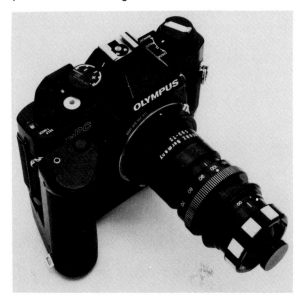

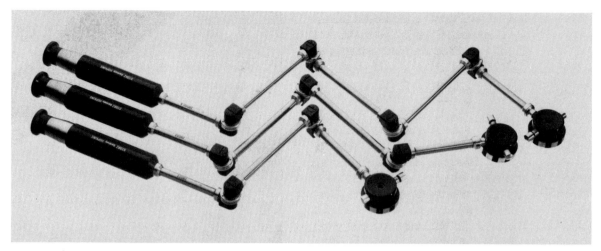

FIG. 3-30. Four-, three-, and two-joint articulated arms. The joints permit optimal movement with no interference to the operator. These teaching arms permit natural color reproduction. A beam splitter can switch the amount of light at the observer's eye from 50% (for examination) to 90% (for documentation).

3. High-resolution viewing monitor. Although television monitors are adequate, their resolution is vastly inferior.
4. Optional: beam splitter that permits either direct viewing through the telescope or indirect viewing of the monitor (Fig. 3-31).

Video photography offers a dynamic arthroscopic view and is an excellent teaching aid. In addition, use of the video monitor enhances the effectiveness of surgical assistants. However, videotapes accumulate rapidly, and storage may become a problem. Furthermore, significant time and cost may be spent on editing. As the arthroscopic skill of the operator improves, he will come to rely more on still photography to illustrate the preoperative and postoperative condition of the joint. With this photographic technique, storage is not a problem and minimal time is invested

FIG. 3-31. Thirty-mm video cameras without beam splitter (*A*) and with beam splitter (*B*). Each camera weighs approximately 50.2 g (1.77 oz).

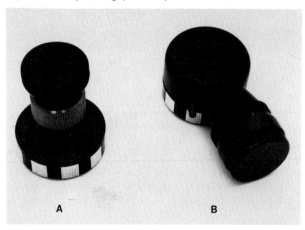

in gathering the documentation (Jackson 1978, Erikson 1979, Shahriaree, Erichsen, 1984).

REFERENCES

Berci G: Instrumenattion 1: Rigid endoscopes. In Berci G: *Endoscopy.* New York, Appleton-Century-Crofts, 1975, pp. 74-112.

Erikson E: Problems in recording arthroscopy. Orthop Clin No Am *10*:735, 1979.

Heffez L, Blaustein DI: Diagnostic arthroscopy of the temporomandibular joint. Part 1: Normal arthroscopic findings. Oral Surg *64*(6): 653–678, 1987.

Jackson DW: Videoarthroscopy: a permanent medical record. Am J Sports Med *6*:213–225, 1978.

Johnson LL, Schneider DA, Austin MD, et al.: Two-percent Gluteraldehyde: A disinfectant in arthroscopy and arthroscopic surgery. J Bone Joint Surg (Am) *64*:237–239, 1982.

Karl Storz Instruction Manual, Katl Storz Endoscopy-America, 1988.

Nemethy G: Instrumentation lll: Cleaning, storage and maintenance and supervision. In Berci G (ed), *Endoscopy*, NY, Appleton-Century-Crofts, 1976, pp. 133–154.

O'Connor RL: *Arthroscopy.* Philadelphia, J B Lippincott Co., 1977, pp. 1–13.

Shahriaree H, Erichsen C: Arthroscopic instrumentation. In Shahriaree H: *O'Connor's Textbook of Arthoscopic Surgery*, Philadelphia, J B Lippincott Co., 1984, pp. 19–35.

Shahriaree H : Recording arthroscopic procedures. In Shahriaree H. *O'Connor's Textbook of Arthroscopic Surgery*, Philadelphia, J B Lippincott Co., 1984, pp. 37–41.

SUGGESTED READINGS

Casscells SW: *Arthroscopy: Diagnostic and Surgical Practice*, Philadelphia, Lea & Febiger, 1984.

DeHaven K: Principles of triangulation for arthroscopic surgery, in Symposium on Arthroscopic Knee Surgery, Orthop Clin No Am *13*:329–336, 1982.

McGinty JB: Closed circuit television in arthroscopy. Rheumatology, *33*:45, 1976.

ARTHROSCOPIC TECHNIQUE

4

The techniques for arthroscopy can be classified according to the space inspected or the number of portals used. Classified by spaces, arthroscopy can be described as superior joint space or inferior joint space arthroscopy. Classified by the number of portals, the technique is described as single-port arthroscopy when only one opening is made into the joint space, or as multiple-port arthroscopy when a second outflow or instrument port is established.

Inferior joint space arthroscopy may be achieved directly via a puncture through the lateral capsule (Murakami, Ono, 1986) or indirectly from the superior space through a perforation of the remodeled retrodiscal tissue (Plate #41). Performing arthroscopy indirectly restricts the field of vision to the area immediately inferior to the perforation. Inferior joint space arthroscopy carries with it the risk of iatrogenic damage to the fibrous and hyaline cartilage surfaces of the condyle. The tight attachments of the medial and lateral capsular ligaments restrict ready access to all recesses of this space.

Only superior space arthroscopy will be discussed here.

PREPARATION FOR ARTHROSCOPY

The particulars of a proper history or physical examination leading to the decision to perform arthroscopy are beyond the scope of this book. The clinical examination preceding the arthroscopic examination and procedure is invaluable. The clinical findings guide the arthroscopist and invariably affect the reported accuracy of the diagnostic arthroscopic examination.

General contraindications to arthroscopy are similar to those for other elective procedures, for example, generalized sepsis or coagulopathies. Markedly restricted mandibular motion owing to ankylosis is a relative contraindication. Clearly, patients with myalgia and no historical or examination findings to support a diagnosis of internal derangement are not candidates for arthroscopy. The orthopedic literature reflects case reports of patients who unfortunately underwent knee arthroscopy for conditions such as Legg-Calvé-Perthes disease and malignant tumors of the femur. The oral and maxillofacial surgeon should select candidates prudently.

The operation is performed with the patient in a supine position with the head resting in a custom foam head holder for stabilization. In thin patients with a good range of cervical motion, the operator may approach both right and left joints from the same side of the operating table. This may be facilitated by having the anesthesiologist tilt the table so that the side of interest approximates the horizontal plane. The field is prepared in the usual sterile manner and draped using an ophthalmologic Steri-drape (3M Surgical Product Division, St. Paul, Minnesota). The external auditory canal is packed with approximately 3 inches of $\frac{1}{4}$ inch iodoform gauze impregnated with bacitracin.

A Mayo stand with arthroscopic instruments (telescopes, trocars, surgical instruments, irrigating syringe, and connecting tubing) is positioned over the patient (Fig. 4-1). A custom-designed instrument holder can suspend the telescopes off the Mayo

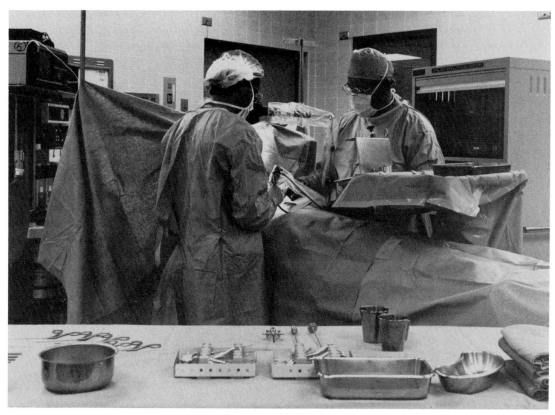

FIG. 4-1. Operator (foreground) and surgical assistant stand at the table. The Mayo stand carrying trocars, surgical instruments, irrigating syringes, and connecting tube is positioned over the patient.

FIG. 4-2. A bird's-eye view of the positioning of the equipment around the operating table. Note the custom-designed arthroscope holder suspended off the Mayo stand. The light-transmitting fiber, video, and TTL cables can be seen running to the video cabinet. The camera with draped articulating arm (arrow) is at the head of the table.

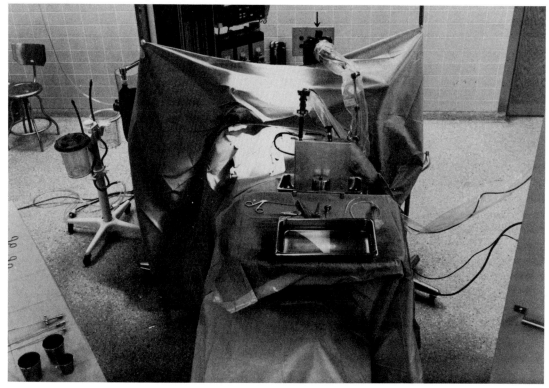

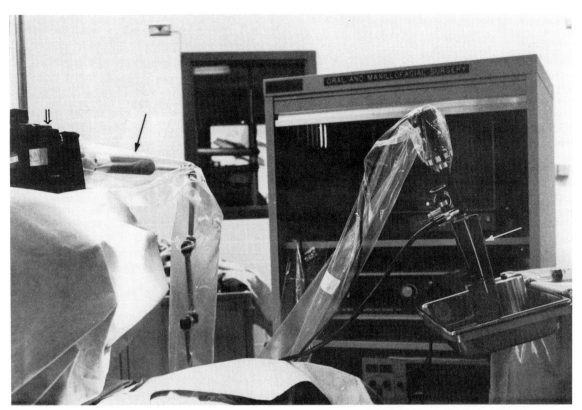

FIG. 4-3. A custom-designed instrument holder (white arrow), fitted to the Mayo stand, suspends the telescopes. The still camera (double arrow) is mounted on a tripod at the head of the table. The articulating arm (black arrow) is draped and may be seen connected to the camera. The mobile cabinet is in the background.

stand, maintaining sterility (the eyepiece is considered nonsterile if viewed directly) and protect the distal working end from being scratched (Figs. 4-2 and 4-3). The operator works more efficiently by being able to reach for the instruments directly rather than having them passed by a nurse assistant. The nurse assistant is positioned on the same side of the table as the operator and behind the Mayo stand. The surgical assistant is positioned in front of the Mayo stand opposite the operator. A mobile cabinet contains the monitor, video transformer, video recorder, and light source (Fig. 4-4). The cabinet may be positioned directly opposite the operator (Figs. 4-5 and 4-6). As mentioned above, in many cases, the operator can perform right and left arthroscopic examinations from the same side of the table. When this is not possible, minor changes in the position of the video cabinet are needed. Some operators may prefer to set the video cabinet at the foot of the operating table (Fig. 4-7). Fiberoptic, TTL photographic, and video camera cables must be long enough to accommodate the extra distance from the patient's head. A foot switch may be used to activate the tape deck.

Still photographic equipment is positioned prior to draping at the head of the table. The camera is mounted on a tripod or on a mechanical arm fastened directly to the side of the operating table (Fig. 3-23). The articulated arm and video camera and cable are draped with sterile sleeves (Arthroscopic Video Camera Drape #1500, Microtek Medical Inc., Columbus, Ohio) (Figs. 4-2 and 4-3) (Heffez, Blaustein, 1987).

SUPERIOR JOINT SPACE PENETRATION

The technique described may be performed with local anesthesia alone, local anesthesia with sedation, or general anesthesia.

Single-port (Fig. 4-8) or two-port systems (Fig. 4-9). may be used in diagnostic arthroscopy. In the single-port system, an outflow cannula is not inserted into the superior joint space; theoretically, a closed circuit system of irrigation exists.

A small towel clamp is inserted at the mandibular angle to assist in the anteroinferior distraction of the mandible. (Fig. 4-10) The location of the condyle is

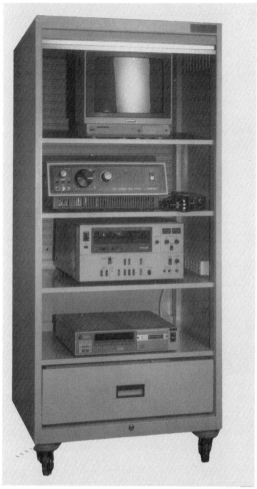

FIG. 4-4. The mobile cabinet containing monitor, light source, ¾-inch video recorder, and ½-inch video recorder.

FIG. 4-5. Standard positioning around the operating table (as seen in Fig. 4-1): operator (1), surgical assistant (2); nurse assistant (3), anesthesiologist (4), patient (triangle), video cabinet (A), Mayo stand (B), accessory instrument table (C).

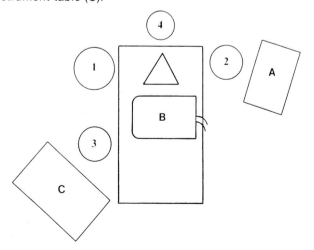

appreciated by moving the mandible and observing its movement subcutaneously, while palpating its lateral pole.

Operators who choose to use a second (outflow) port may begin with its insertion. The outflow cannula should be inserted anterior and inferior to the apex of the anterior tubercle. The incision will usually lie approximately 15 mm anterior to the tragus, and 1 to 2 cm anterior and inferior to the articular eminence (Figs. 4-10 and 4-11).

Placement of the stab incision for the outflow cannula immediately inferior, rather than anteroinferior, to the tubercle will cause scuffing of the fibrous connective tissue covering of the eminence when the joint space is penetrated. The incision for the outflow port is made through skin and subcutaneous tissue using a #11 blade. A mosquito hemostat is used to undermine the skin edges and then to bluntly dissect toward the anterior tubercle. Once this structure is appreciated with the tips of the hemostat, the outflow cannula with its sharp trocar is inserted and directed posterosuperiorly to contact the anterior tubercle (Figs. 4-10 and 4-12). The cannula-trocar unit is then backed off the tubercle and directed immediately anterior to this structure, in order to penetrate the anterior recess of the superior joint space.

The incision for the inflow port (sheath) is located posterior to the incision for the outflow port. The incision for the inflow port should be traced now in order to ensure that approximately 1.5 cm of bridging tissue exists between incisions (Fig. 4-9B). This permits optimum movement of the telescope without interfering with the outflow cannula. The landmarks for incision placement are the anterior tubercle, and the lateral aspect of the glenoid fossa and condyle (Fig. 4-12). The incision for placement of the telescope is traced as a 1- to 2-mm vertical line perpendicular to the outline of the lateral rim of the glenoid fossa and over its presumed region of highest concavity. The incision usually falls approximately 5 mm anterior to the tragus of the ear. Preoperative open mouth radiographs may assist in planning this incision. From these films, the operator may note the relationship of the posterolateral aspect of the condyle to the region of highest contour of the glenoid fossa. Incisions are better located too low than too high when ease of joint penetration alone is considered. A stab incision is made and the skin edges undermined to minimize traumatic abrasion during the arthroscopic examination. The superior joint space is then entered, via the incision, using a 19-gauge needle attached to a 5-ml syringe. The joint space is dilated with either an epinephrine or a lactated Ringer's solution. Lactated Ringer's solution is preferred because it does

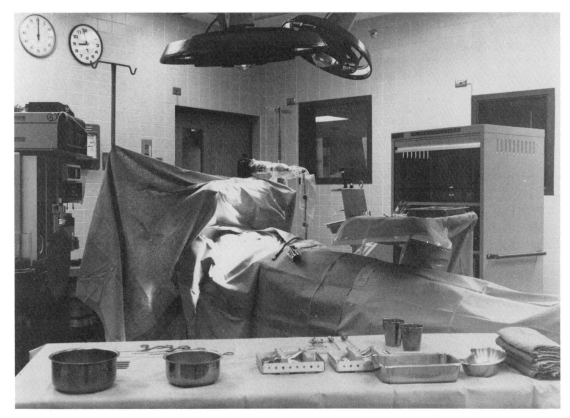

FIG. 4-6. Positioning of the equipment around the operating table.

FIG. 4-7. Alternative positioning: operator (1), surgical assistant (2), nurse assistant (3), anesthesiologist (4), patient (triangle), video cabinet (A), Mayo stand (B), and accessory instrument table (C).

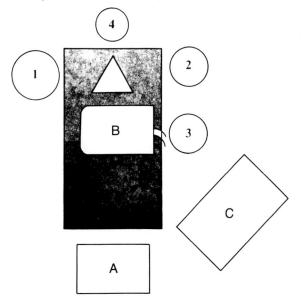

not interfere with the evaluation of the superficial vascularity of the retrodiscal and remodeled retrodiscal tissues. The needle is inserted in an inferosuperior direction, at an angle of 5 to 10 degrees to the skin surface, in order to contact the lateral rim of the glenoid fossa (Fig. 4-13). Once this structure is contacted, the needle is guided or "walked" inferiorly and medially, with the assistance of the index finger of the contralateral hand. The goal is to negotiate around the lateral rim of the glenoid fossa until the concavity of the glenoid fossa is felt. Joint dilation is then accomplished with 1 to 2 ml of irrigant, and the 19-gauge needle is withdrawn.

Attention is now directed to penetration of the joint space with the trocar and sheath (Fig. 4-14). The capsule and lateral temporomandibular ligament are approached through the first incision with blunt dissection using a mosquito hemostat. The operator may verify the position of the hemostat by having the assistant distract the mandible in an anterior and inferior direction, while the instrument is held against the lateral capsule.

A sharp trocar, locked to the 2.7-mm sheath to form a single unit, is grasped between index and major fingers and thumb (Fig. 4-15). This grasp permits op-

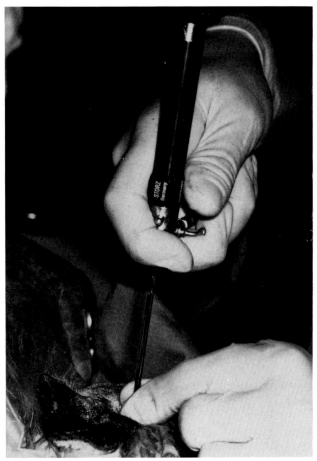

FIG. 4-8. Cranial view of single-port arthroscopy of a live baboon.

timum control of the instrument. Three factors facilitate lateral entry into the superior joint space: the tendency of gravity to tilt the jaw inferomedially owing to muscle relaxation and horizontal positioning of the head, dilation of the space with a fluid medium, and active distraction of the mandible in an anterior and inferior direction by the assistant. Frequently, active distraction is not required. Penetration of the superior joint space of bulbous condyles has proven the most difficult, requiring that all three of the previously mentioned factors be operative. Yale et al. (1966) identified four basic condyle shapes in a series of 3008 dried condyles. They described the incidence of bulbous condyles as 3%.

The technique of penetration with the sharp trocar is identical with the technique used to penetrate the joint space with the 19-gauge needle used for joint space distension. Once the region of greatest concavity is appreciated, the unit is held against the posterior slope of the eminence/ roof of the glenoid fossa

with thumb and index finger of the contralateral hand (Fig. 4-16). The sharp trocar is removed from the sheath, and the workhorse of arthroscopy, the 2.4-mm 30 degree forward-oblique viewing telescope, inserted. Whenever a change to telescope or trocar is required, the unit is positioned gently against the bone of the glenoid fossa to ensure that medial penetration of the joint cavity does not occur. The arthroscopic examination is performed under dilation provided by lactated Ringer's solution to maintain hemostasis and increase the volume of the superior joint space sufficiently to permit adequate examination. For this purpose, an extension tube is connected to the stopcock of the sheath and a 50-ml syringe (Fig. 4-17). Lactated Ringer's solution is preferred over saline because the pH of normal saline is more variable and slightly acidic, at pH 5.3. In addition, saline solution in volumes greater than 500 ml has been noted to reduce proteoglycan synthesis by chondrocytes (Reagen et al., 1983). Gas arthroscopy using carbon dioxide or nitrogen has been used extensively by European orthopedic colleagues (Eriksson, Sebik, 1982). Ohnishi (1980) reported the use of gas arthroscopy in temporomandibular joint arthroscopy.

A diagnostic examination may usually be completed within 10 to 15 minutes using 30 to 50 ml of irrigant. Suction may be applied continuously to an outflow cannula, or the irrigant can simply be allowed to accumulate within a fold in the disposable drape and then suctioned intermittently.

In single-port arthroscopy, quantities of fluid exceeding 250 ml have been injected with no permanent side effects noted. Some of the fluid refluxes out of the joint space along the sheath. Experience gained with computed tomography with double contrast arthrography reveals that the remainder of the fluid travels medially into the pterygomandibular and infratemporal spaces as well as posterosuperiorly and laterally along the neck of the condyle (Heffez et al., 1988). This accumulation of fluid may be responsible for transient paresthesias of the inferior alveolar and lingual nerves. In our experience, operators find that the outflow port unnecessarily crowds the operative site and interferes with the diagnostic examination. The single-port system, by virtue of being more of a closed system, may provide greater dilation of the superior joint space and thus improved hemostasis. Insertion of an outflow cannula increases the danger of injuring the facial zygomatic nerve, located 8 to 32 mm anterior to the anterior margin of the bony external auditory canal (Al Kayat, Bramley, 1979). There is also increased danger of damaging the telescopic lens if *triangulation* is not mastered. Triangulation is the technique by which the telescope and instrument/

FIG. 4-9. Two-port arthroscopy. *A*, A second anterior eminence port may be used during both diagnostic and surgical arthroscopy. *B*, A second inferior port is used during surgical arthroscopy for manipulation of instruments in the inferior space.

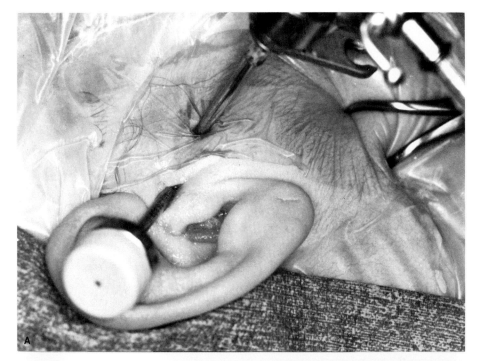

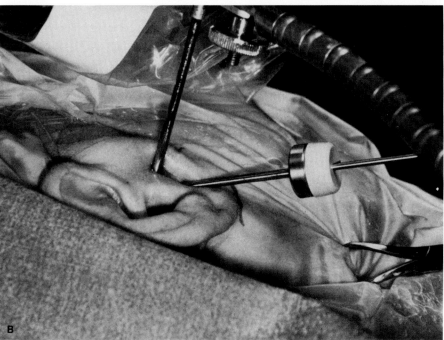

suction are manipulated from outside the joint space, to directly visualize the instrument or to allow for continuous outflow of the irrigation fluid (Fig. 4-9A,B) (DeHaven, 1982). Some authors choose to reserve the term triangulation for the manipulation of three separate instruments through three ports and the term biangulation for the manipulation of two instruments (DeHaven, 1982). A malleable tension arm may assist in holding the telescope while a second instrument

is manipulated through the second port (Fig. 3-23; Fig. 4-18).

We recommend completing the diagnostic examination with the single-port system, inserting an outflow cannula if visibility is obscured by debris or if surgical arthroscopy is indicated. With insertion of the second port, the operator may choose to alternate inflow (telescope) and outflow sites depending on the arthroscopic procedure contemplated. When trian-

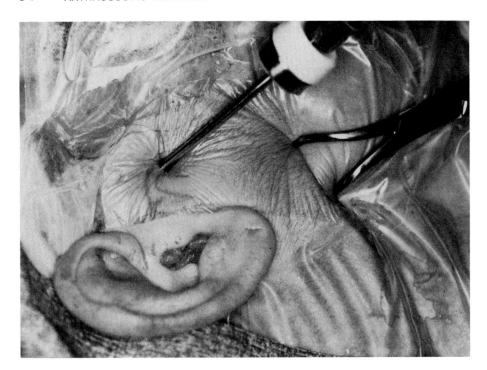

gulation is performed, a mechanical flexible arm may be used for stabilization of the arthroscope.

Systematic complete examination of the superior joint space is done by observing the joint space on the video monitor or directly through the telescope. (Heffez, Blaustein, 1987)

ARTHROSCOPIC ANATOMIC NOMENCLATURE

The arthroscopic nomenclature for normal anatomic structures is described below. The arthroscopic nomenclature for pathologic structures is described in Chapter 6. The term posterior incline of the posterior band is used to describe the posterior, upward slope of the posterior band (Fig. 4-19). Anterior incline of the posterior band refers to the anterior, downward slope of the posterior band (Fig. 4-19). The crest of the posterior band refers to the peak of the posterior band. It occurs at the junction of the posterior and anterior inclines (Fig. 4-19). The term lateral sulcus is used to describe the groove formed by the reflection of the lateral capsule onto the lateral edge

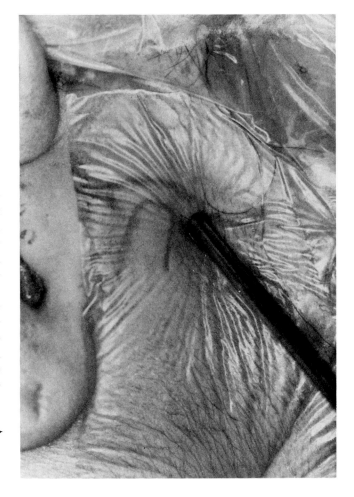

FIG. 4-11. An instrument has been inserted through the sheath of the second port; the instrument and sheath have been manipulated into the glenoid regions.

FIG. 4-12. The landmarks are traced: anterior tubercle, lateral aspect of the glenoid fossa, and condyle.

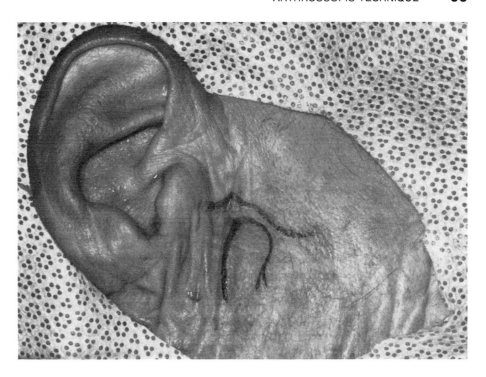

of the disc (Fig. 4-20). The term medial sulcus is used to describe the groove formed by the reflection of the medial capsule onto the lateral edge of the disc (Fig. 4-20). The flexure in the normal condyle-disc-fossa relationship represents the junction of the tympanic portion of the retrodiscal tissue with the posterior incline of the posterior band (Fig. 4-19, Plate 1). A knife-edged prolongation of the synovium covering the articular surface of the posterior attachment over the posterior band may be noted anterior to the flexure. These superficial transversely oriented synovial vessels should not be confused with the vessels found

FIG. 4-13. The 19-gauge needle is directed inferosuperiorly at an angle of 5 to 10 degrees to the skin surface, to contact the lateral rim of the glenoid fossa. The needle is then "walked" around the rim inferiorly and medially, to contact the greatest concavity of the glenoid fossa.

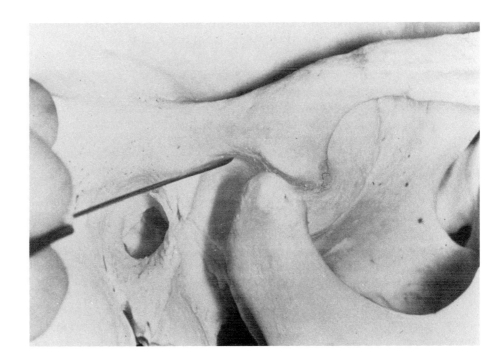

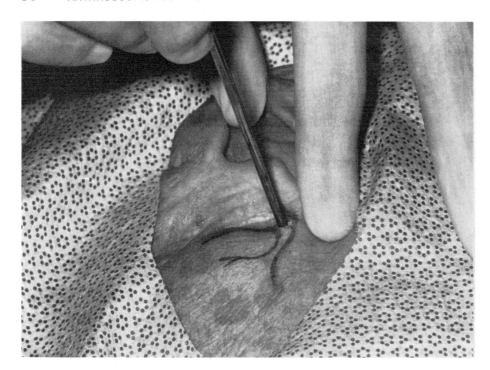

FIG. 4-14. Penetration of the superior joint space with sharp trocar and sheath.

within the substance of remodeled retrodiscal tissue. The former appear to be present in a thin translucent membrane overlying another structure.

Murakami and Hoshino (1982) described an arthroscopic nomenclature using terms such as anterior and posterior pouches and higher and lower intermediate spaces. We prefer to use regional nomenclature based on osseous landmarks because pathologic and postsurgical conditions may make identification of soft-tissue landmarks difficult and because radi-

ographs offer a convenient blueprint of the joint. Osseous remodeling changes tend to parallel soft-tissue changes at a slower rate.

That portion of the superior joint space located under the concavity of the glenoid fossa is called the *glenoid region* (Fig. 4-21). It is bounded posteriorly by the attachment of the tympanic portion of the retrodiscal tissue and anteriorly by the apex of the eminence. The glenoid region is divided into *anterior* and *posterior glenoid regions* by an imaginary vertical plane dropped from the area of maximum concavity of the glenoid fossa. This concavity is a convenient landmark, as it is a natural resting point for the telescope. The *pre-eminence region* represents that portion of the superior joint space bounded posteriorly by the apex of the eminence and anteriorly by the anterior and anteromedial capsule (Fig. 4-21). The apex of the eminence is readily recognized arthroscopically (Heffez, Blaustein, 1987).

EXAMINATION OF THE SUPERIOR JOINT SPACE

Following the puncture of the superior joint space and introduction of the telescope, the operator first establishes that the telescope is indeed positioned in a space, so not to mistakenly identify extracapsular structures as intracapsular ones.

FIG. 4-15. Grasping the sheath between index and major fingers and thumb assures optimum control.

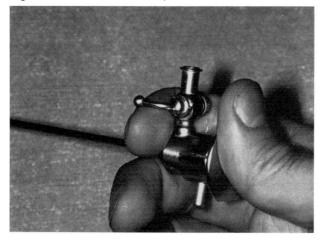

FIG. 4-16. During a change of instruments, the sheath is held firmly but gently against the roof of the glenoid fossa with the thumb and index fingers.

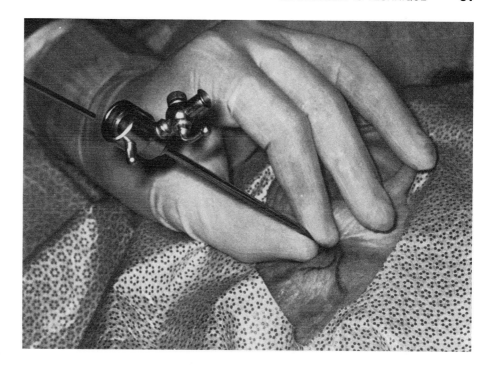

Six parameters are used to judge location and formulate an accurate diagnosis—color, surface morphology, texture, orientation of structures, joint space configuration, and topographic relationships. For instance, the disc is stark white, remodeled retrodiscal tissue is yellow-white or ivory, with variable degrees of superficial vascularity, normal retrodiscal tissue, is pink, and medial and lateral ligaments are gray. The smooth, regular surface of the disc contrasts with the irregular surface of the remodeled retrodiscal tissue. Texturally, the firm, compact disc contrasts with the soft, pliable retrodiscal tissue. Orientation of structures can aid in diagnosis; for instance, the tympanic portion of the retrodiscal tissue, shows a vertical an-

FIG. 4-17. Extension tube connected to the stopcock on the 2.7 mm external sheath.

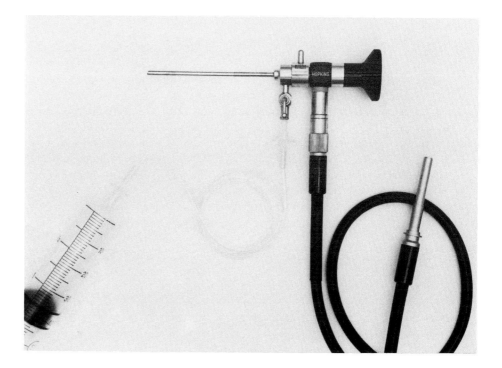

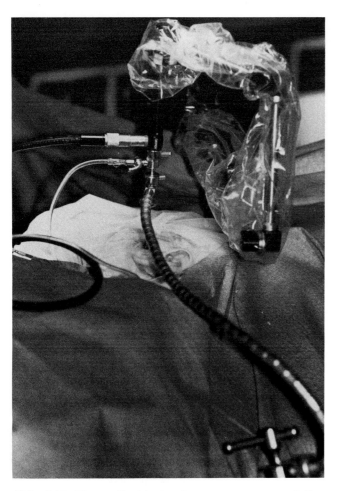

FIG. 4-18. The malleable tension arm can support the weight of the telescope and video camera and can facilitate triangulation.

gulation, whereas the remodeled retrodiscal tissue shows a horizontal angulation. Joint space configuration can also help, such as the posteroinferior to anterosuperior orientation of the joint space over the posterior incline of the posterior band (Fig. 4-22). Topographic relationships are also significant, such as the anterior incline of the posterior band related to the termination of the medial capsular ligament.

TECHNIQUE

Initially, a sweeping motion is employed with the telescope in order to assimilate several fields of view. The junction of the posterior attachment of the retrodiscal tissue with the posterior band serves as the principal orientation landmark in the normal con-

dyle-disc-fossa relationship (Plate 1). This landmark is referred to as the flexure because of its V or U configuration. This flexure landmark is artificially exaggerated by the introduction of the telescope and irrigation fluid. Sagittal histologic specimens of the temporomandibular joint in an open mouth position reveal the nature of the flexure (Fig. 1-2). Preparation of the specimen causes some shrinkage of the tissues, and thus the relationships observed mimic the structural relationships noted under arthroscopy. The artefacts created in the arthroscopic examination are revealed with examination of magnetic resonance images. The superior joint space is a virtual space. With any degree of opening, the vessels within the retrodiscal tissue engorge with blood to such an extent that the retrodiscal tissue and remodeled retrodiscal tissue can be seen to expand to approximate the temporal bone (Fig. 1-21).

One means of identifying the flexure without causing iatrogenic trauma is to gently direct the telescope posteriorly in the direction of the external auditory canal (Fig. 4-23A, B). In this way, the telescope is in the appropriate geographic position to observe the flexure and a specific orientation coordinate is thus established.

In normal disc relationships the flexure may be recognized by looking for abrupt color and orientation changes. At the flexure, the pink, vertical or oblique retrodiscal tissue, bearing a few surface vessels, joins with the stark white tissue of the posterior incline of the posterior band. Typically, several transversely oriented surface vessels of the posterior attachment are seen in the region of the flexure (Plate 7). In the displaced disc, the flexure is formed by the junction between the tympanic portion of the retrodiscal tissue and the remodeled retrodiscal tissue overlying the condyle (Plate 12). The flexure appears more U shaped in the normal to slightly displaced disc position and more V shaped in the moderate to severely anteriorly displaced disc (see Chapter 6). On microscopic examination the flexure represents only a small field in comparison to the rest of the superior joint space (see Chapter 1). The arthroscopist must remember that the telescope magnifies the anatomic details. At 1-mm distance, an object is magnified approximately ten times. At 1-cm distance, no magnification occurs.

EXAMINATION PHASES

There are three examination phases: transverse, longitudinal, and dynamic transverse.

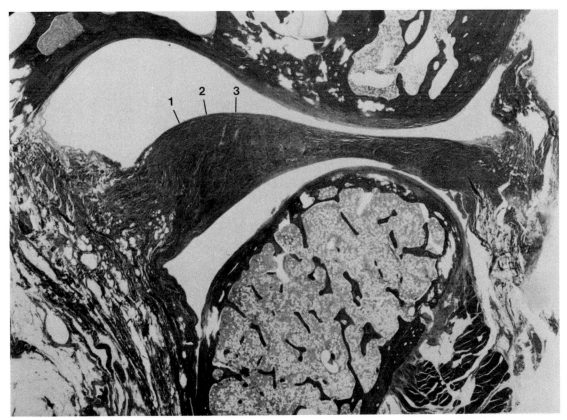

FIG. 4-19. Right TMJ sagittal microscopic section. Note the posterior incline (1), crest (2), and anterior incline (3) of the posterior band.

Transverse Phase

This phase of the arthroscopic examination is used for evaluation of the glenoid fossa and the tissues immediately beneath it (anterior and posterior glenoid regions). The telescope is moved along the transverse plane of the superior joint space. The correct orientation of the telescope is indicated in Figure 4-24A,B. This portion of the examination provides information about the nature of the flexure, vascularity of the tympanic portion of the retrodiscal tissue and remodeled tissues, irregularities in the glenoid fossa, integrity of the medial capsule and ligament, and position of the posterior band.

Longitudinal Phase

This phase of the arthroscopic examination is used to evaluate the tissues lying anterior to the apex of the eminence. The telescope is moved along the longitudinal axis of the superior joint space, the operator

FIG. 4-20. Illustration demonstrating the lateral (1) and medial (2) sulci of the superior joint space.

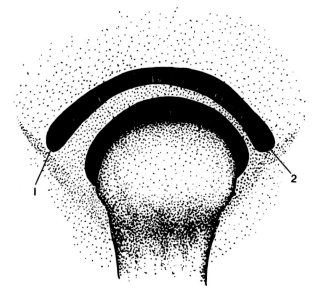

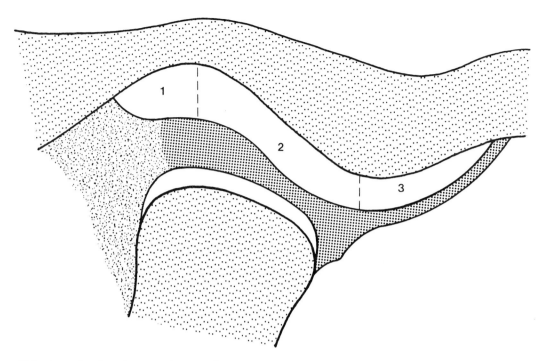

FIG. 4-21. Regional anatomic classification is based on osseous landmarks. The superior joint space is divided into posterior glenoid (1), anterior glenoid (2), and pre-eminence (3) regions. Vertical planes drawn from the region of maximum concavity of the glenoid fossa and apex of the eminence serve as the boundaries.

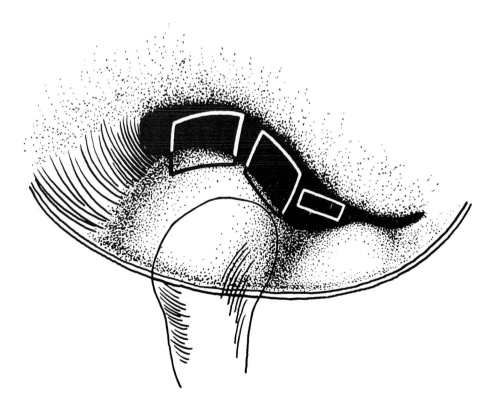

FIG. 4-22. Illustration of a right TMJ depicting the change in direction and configuration of the superior joint space. Note the posteroinferior to anterosuperior inclination over the posterior incline of the posterior band; the posterosuperior to anteroinferior inclination over the anterior incline of the posterior band; and the parallelogram over the intermediate zone.

FIG. 4-23. The flexure (arrow) is identified by orienting the telescope toward the external auditory canal. An angiocatheter is used to simulate the endoscope. *B*, Close-up view of the angiocatheter in place.

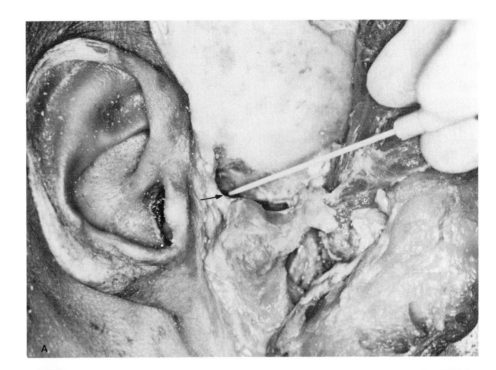

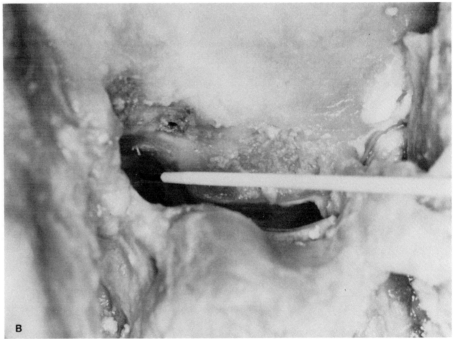

recording findings per arthroscopic field. The correct orientation of the telescope is indicated in Figure 4-25. In disc displacements, this portion of the examination permits the operator to confirm the position of the stark white remodeled disc anterior to the mandibular condyle; identify the junction of the remodeled retrodiscal tissue with remodeled disc; verify the integrity of the anterior portion of the lateral capsule

ligament and medial capsule; and comment on surface irregularities in the fibrous covering of the eminence and remodeled retrodiscal tissues.

Dynamic Transverse Phase

This phase is performed while holding the telescope and sheath along the transverse axis of the su-

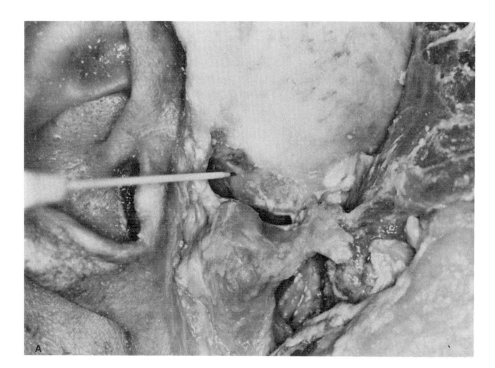

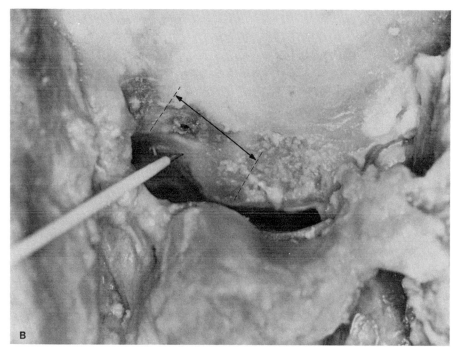

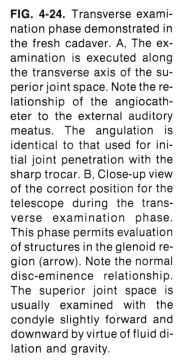

FIG. 4-24. Transverse examination phase demonstrated in the fresh cadaver. A, The examination is executed along the transverse axis of the superior joint space. Note the relationship of the angiocatheter to the external auditory meatus. The angulation is identical to that used for initial joint penetration with the sharp trocar. B, Close-up view of the correct position for the telescope during the transverse examination phase. This phase permits evaluation of structures in the glenoid region (arrow). Note the normal disc-eminence relationship. The superior joint space is usually examined with the condyle slightly forward and downward by virtue of fluid dilation and gravity.

perior joint space and having the assistant gently move the mandible backward and forward. This portion of the examination permits the operator to comment on the filling of the superficial vessels of the remodeled retrodiscal tissue during simulated opening and closing, stretching of the retrodiscal tissue, and location of the load-bearing zone during translation.

PROCEDURE

The transverse examination phase is performed first because the technique for penetration of the joint space calls for placement of the trocar, the sheath, and then the telescope along its transverse axis. More medial and central fields of the joint space are inspected before proceeding to the lateral aspects. Ex-

FIG. 4-25. Longitudinal examination phase executed in the fresh cadaver. The telescope is oriented along the longitudinal axis of the superior joint space so that joint structures in the pre-eminence region (arrow) can be evaluated.

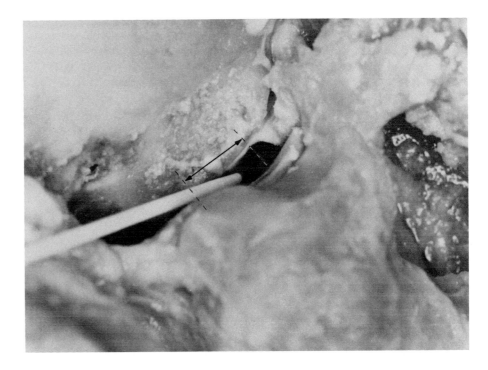

amination is performed in this manner because the telescope/sheath may slip out of the joint space during lateral examinations. In some cases, positioning the mandible posteriorly will allow the telescope to roll over into the anterior fields. At the conclusion of this examination phase, the operator proceeds to the longitudinal examination phase.

The sheath and telescope are gently but firmly positioned on the roof of the glenoid fossa. The telescope is removed and replaced with the blunt trocar (Fig. 4-16). The trocar and sheath are then moved, as a unit, beyond the apex of the eminence and into the pre-eminence region. This movement is most easily accomplished by walking the trocar/sheath unit around the lateral aspect of the eminence and then directing it anteromedially. In performing this maneuver, the clinician must keep in mind the axis of the eminence. The telescope will usually enter the medial aspect of the pre-eminence region, because the attachment of the lateral capsular ligament makes it difficult to distract the condyle in an anterior direction. It must be remembered that the medial capsular ligament terminates, abruptly, in the glenoid region. If the instrument is directed medially with too much force, the medial capsule may be perforated. The operator may find the examination more easily performed if the assistant distracts the condyle inferiorly (not anteroinferiorly). In many cases, joint laxity permits the operator to move directly from the transverse examination phase to the longitudinal phase without removing the telescope. The technique

used for entering the pre-eminence region under direct vision is the same as that described above. The operator then completes the examination by performing the dynamic phase.

The telescope/sheath usually slips back easily into the transverse axis of the joint space when it is gently withdrawn from the pre-eminence region. A change of instruments is not needed. In order for the operator to assess disc relationships, the assistant should make a conscious effort to reposition the condyle posterosuperiorly in the glenoid fossa. The positioning of the patient's head, muscle relaxation, and joint space dilation cause the mandible to move, unassisted, in an anteroinferior direction. This movement may give the operator a false impression of disc relationships. The assistant then gently distracts the mandible backward and forward, while the operator assesses the condition of the tissues.

During each phase of the examination the arthroscopic findings are systematically logged. A sample arthroscopic log is shown in Figure 4-26.

Arthroscopic findings of the transverse examination phase are recorded. The region under the glenoid fossa is divided into a grid consisting of nine overlapping arthroscopic fields. The grid system is formed by the intersection of three transverse regions—anterior, middle, and posterior—and three parasagittal regions—lateral, central, and medial. An arthroscopic field in question is located by describing the transverse-parasagittal coordinates (Fig. 4-27). For example, an arthroscopic field is described as Posterior-medial and traditionally abbreviated as P_m (Fig. 4-27). The middle-central field corresponds to the field approximating the region of highest concavity of the glenoid fossa. The flexure is found in the posterior fields. The posterior slope of the eminence is seen in the anterior fields.

In the longitudinal examination phase, arthroscopic findings are recorded according to three fields oriented transversely: lateral, central, and medial.

With completion of the three phases of the examination, the telescope is withdrawn, without removing the sheath from the joint space. In the single-port system, irrigation fluid and any debris within the superior joint space are suctioned using a Frazier suction tip passed blindly through the sheath. The sheath is then removed. In the two-port system, the superior space is irrigated until the fluid from the outflow port appears clear. The sheath and cannula are then removed. Skin is closed with a single 5-0 nylon suture, and Steristrips (3M Surgical Product Division, St Paul, Minnesota) are placed. Placement of the suture maintains wound closure in the presence of drainage through the puncture wounds over the first 24 hours of joint function. Antibiotics are not routinely prescribed, and corticosteroids are not routinely injected post-arthroscopy. An arthroscopic log is completed immediately on termination of the examination if it has not been completed during the procedure (Heffez, Blaustein, 1987.)

POSTOPERATIVE CARE

Physical therapy is an integral part of diagnostic and surgical arthroscopy. The patient's failure to comply with home physiotherapeutic exercises may result in fibrous ankylosis. The patient is informed that persistent leakage of blood-tinged fluid from the puncture sites is normal for the first 24 hours of joint function. Blood clots that may be trapped in the external auditory canal can be loosened with gentle irrigation with normal saline. Invariably these clots will loosen and be expelled from the canal over several weeks. Should the attendant decrease in hearing annoy the patient, the surgeon may irrigate the external auditory canal with peroxide/normal saline solution to dislodge the clots.

Exercises are prescribed to increase the range of joint motion. The patient is cautioned to perform the exercises gently, never strenuously. If the exercises

FIG. 4-26. The arthroscopic log.

Date _____

Patient Name _____
Hospital Number _____
Address _____
_____

Telephone _____ bus.
_____ home

KEY

mf / lf	medial/lateral folds
v	vessels
rdt	remodeled retrodiscal tissue
rdt	retrodiscal tissue
d	disc
p	perforations
A_w	adhesions: weblike
A_l	linear bands
sp	synovial plica
fb	foreign body
t	tears of fibrous connective tissue
f	fibrillation
——	other findings

I. TRANSVERSE EXAMINATION PHASE

Flexure identified   yes / no

ORIENT ARTHROSCOPIC MAP BELOW AND INDICATE FINDINGS USING KEY

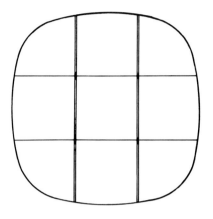

Comments: _____
_____
_____
_____

II. LONGITUDINAL EXAMINATION PHASE

Junction of remodeled retrodiscal tissue and disc identified: yes / no

ORIENT ARTHROSCOPIC MAP BELOW AND INDICATE FINDINGS USING KEY

COMMENTS _____
_____
_____

III. DYNAMIC TRANSVERSE PHASE

Condyle pressing on remodeled retrodiscal tissue?   yes / no

Comments _____
_____
_____

ARTHROSCOPIC DIAGNOSIS _____
_____

FIG. 4-26. (Continued)

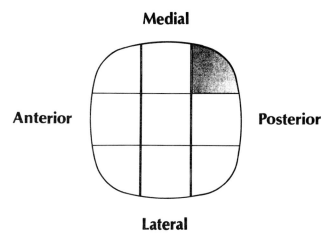

Medial

Anterior

Posterior

Lateral

FIG. 4-27. Arthroscopic findings in the transverse examination phase are recorded according to the field of view in which they are observed. The glenoid fossa is divided into a grid consisting of nine components. The shaded field represents the Posterior-medial field (P_m).

cause undue pain, they should be discontinued for a brief time, then gradually repeated. Typically three types of exercises may be prescribed: an opening stretching exercise, a protrusion exercise, and a combination protrusion and opening exercise. Only the first two exercises are performed during the first 2 postoperative weeks. The third exercise may be prescribed if the patient has not gained a satisfactory range of motion, which is considered as greater than 30 mm of opening, by the 2-week interval.

The patient begins with five repetitions of each exercise and increases this to twenty. The entire sequence is repeated 3 times a day. The patient is encouraged to progress to diets of increasing consistency and to chew sugarless gum.

Most patients will respond to this simple home exercise program. In some cases, the assistance of a physical therapist is needed.

LIMITS OF THE EXAMINATION

Most of the anatomic relationships of the superior joint space may be readily inspected arthroscopically. The technique for examining the pre-eminence region is the most difficult to master. The infratemporal articulating surface, upward sloping of the intermediate zone (anterior band), and anterior capsule may thus escape observation. The lateral attachment of the capsule to the disc in the glenoid region, being the site of penetration of the telescope, cannot be seen. When a second more anterior port is used and the telescope introduced through that port, the operator is still unable to appreciate this lateral capsular attachment because of the angulation of the telescope.

Perforations of the remodeled retrodiscal tissue, present on arthrography, have not always been identified arthroscopically. Although the possibility always exists that the perforations were iatrogenic, the skill of the arthrographic technique has been mastered. Williams and Laskin (1980) and Liedberg and Westesson (1986) also found it difficult to confirm the presence of perforations during arthroscopy. The latter authors found that arthroscopy provided high reliability and low sensitivity when it came to diagnosing internal derangements in fresh cadavers. However, Holmlund and Hellsing (1985) reported 100% arthroscopic accuracy for diagnosing arthrotic changes in block autopsy specimens of the TMJ. While fresh cadaver specimens remain the optimum model for teaching arthroscopy, the superficial vascularity and fibrillar nature of tissues are difficult to appreciate except in the living patient. The gross delineation of remodeled retrodiscal tissue and disc is not simple. Isaacson et al. (1986) commented on the decrease in vascularity of the remodeled retrodiscal tissue as contributing to a surgical misdiagnosis. Diagnostic arthroscopy may ease this confusion.

We have performed only indirect arthroscopy of the inferior joint space (Plate 41). Regular examination of this joint space is precluded by the tight attachments of the lateral and medial capsular ligaments to the disc and condyle, proximity of the fibrocartilage of the condyle, and narrowness of the joint space. The effects of iatrogenic arthroscopic injury to the condylar cartilage have yet to be fully assessed.

REFERENCES

Al-Kayat A, Bramley P: A modified preauricular approach to the temporomandibular joint and malar arch. Br J Oral Surg 17:91–103, 1979.

DeHaven K: Principles of triangulation for arthroscopic surgery, in Symposium on Arthroscopic Knee Surgery, Orthop Clin No Am 13:329–336, 1982.

Eriksson E, Sebik A: Arthroscopy and arthroscopic surgery in a gas versus a fluid medium. Symposium on arthroscopic knee surgery. Orthop Clin No Am 13:293–298, 1982.

Heffez L, Blaustein DI: Diagnostic arthroscopy of the temporomandibular joint. Part 1: Normal arthroscopic findings. Oral Surg 64(6):653–678, 1987.

Heffez L, Mafee MF, Langer B: Double contrast arthrography of the temporomandibular joint: Role of direct sagittal CT imaging. Oral Surg 65:511–514, 1988.

Holmlund A, Hellsing G: Arthroscopy of the temporomandibular joint. An autopsy study. Int J Oral Surg 14:169-175, 1985.

Isaacson G, Isberg A, Johansson AS et al.: Internal derangement of the temporomandibular joint: Radiographic and histologic changes associated with severe pain. J Oral Maxillofac Surg *44*:771–778, 1986.

Liedberg J, Westesson PL: Diagnostic accuracy of upper compartment arthroscopy of the temporomandibular joint. Correlation with postmortem morphology. Oral Surg *62*(6):618–24, 1986.

Murakami K, Hashino K: Regional anatomical nomenclature and arthroscopic terminology in human temporomandibular joints. Okajimas Folla Anat Jpn *58*:745–760, 1982.

Murakami K, Ono T: Temporomandibular joint arthroscopy by inferolateral approach. Int J Oral Maxillofac Surg *15*:410–417, 1986.

Ohnishi M: Clinical application of arthroscopy in the temporomandibular joint diseases. Bull Tokyo Med Dent Univ *27*:141–150, 1980.

Reagan BF, McInerny VK, Treadwell BV, et al. Irrigating solutions for arthroscopy. J Bone Joint Surg *65*-A:629–631, 1983.

Williams RA, Laskin DM: Arthroscopic examination of experimentally induced pathologic conditions of the rabbit temporomandibular joint. J Oral Surg *38*:652–659, 1980.

Yale SH, Allison BD, Hauptfuehrer JD: An epidemiological assessment of mandibular condyle morphology, Oral Surg *21*:169–177, 1966.

SUGGESTED READINGS

Jackson RW, Dandy DJ: *Arthroscopy of the Knee*. New York, Grune & Stratton, 1976.

O'Connor RL: *Arthroscopy*. Philadelphia, JB Lippincott Co., 1977.

Shahriaree H, Erichsen C: Arthroscopic instrumentation. In Shahriaree H: *O'Connor's Textbook of Arthroscopic Surgery*, Philadelphia, J B Lippincott Co, 1984, pp 19–35.

Shahriaree Heshmat: *O'Connor's Textbook of Arthroscopic Surgery*. Philadelphia, JB Lippincott Co, 1984

NORMAL ARTHROSCOPIC ANATOMY

5

The criteria for normal arthroscopic anatomy were established by correlating horizontally and vertically corrected arthrotomograms and/ or direct gross intra-articular examination with arthroscopic examinations, of primarily fresh and embalmed cadaver temporomandibular joints (Heffez, Blaustein, 1987). Only a few arthroscopic examinations have been performed on the live patient with normal disc relationships.

The arthroscopic findings are described below according to each of the examination phases. In each field of view, the arthroscopist must check color, surface morphology, texture, orientation of structures, joint space configuration, and topographic relationships. The accuracy of diagnostic arthroscopy depends on the meticulous technique of the operator.

The text is referenced with plates selected from those at the end of the chapter.

TRANSVERSE EXAMINATION PHASE

The arthroscopic findings during this phase are described according to their location in the posterior, middle, or anterior fields. In general, all of the medial fields of the superior joint space are examined first, followed by the central fields, and lastly by the lateral fields. This method helps avoid premature withdrawal from the joint space.

The anatomic relationships can be fully appreciated only if the findings in all of the arthroscopic fields are correlated. The operator might need to move the telescope back into a field of view already examined to confirm certain impressions. Rotating the telescope

in place greatly increases the field of vision and permits closer examination of structures (Fig. 3-9).

POSTERIOR-MEDIAL (P$_m$), POSTERIOR-CENTRAL (P$_c$), AND POSTERIOR-LATERAL (P$_l$) FIELDS

Anatomic structures readily identified in these fields include retrodiscal tissue, posterior attachment, posterior incline of the posterior band, synovium of the glenoid fossa, posterior aspect of the medial sulcus, synovial plicae, and medial capsule.

Posteromedially, the retrodiscal tissue is oriented obliquely in a superior to inferior direction to attach anteriorly to the stark white posterior band via the posterior attachment (Plate 1). Folds (pleats) (usually two) in the tympanic portion of the retrodiscal tissue have been noted in the fresh cadaver. The folds are labeled as medial and lateral folds. The existence of folds in the normal TMJ of the live patient has not yet been established. However, their existence in the internally deranged joint is common (Plate 14).

The region of the posterior attachment is more easily recognized in the middle and lateral fields where usually three to five vessels course transversally (Plates 6 and 7). The retrodiscal tissue may appear pink to off-white. Typically a few surface vessels are seen coursing randomly. The fibrous connective tissue of the roof of the glenoid fossa is ivory white with only an occasional blood vessel visible. A number of synovial vessels course superiorly from the medial sulcus. These vessels appear to terminate a short distance from the medial sulcus (Plate 3). The tissue colors of the synovium (ivory), retrodiscal tissue (pink), and posterior band (stark white) are distinguishing features.

The posterior aspect of the gray to ivory medial capsular ligament is visible. During arthroscopic examination, with the condyle distracted anteroinferiorly by fluid dilation, the medial capsular ligament fibers are oriented posteroinferior to anterosuperior (Plate 9). With increasing condylar translation, the ligament's fibers of insertion move anteriorly, and thus the orientation of the ligament changes from posterosuperior to anteroinferior. A synovial plica can be seen in the most posterior region of the medial sulcus (Plate 4). The plica is usually smooth and has several small surface vessels. A bulbous condyle may prevent observation of this region.

Posterocentrally and posterolaterally, the retrodiscal tissue appears to be oriented more vertically (Plate 7), and more of the glenoid fossa is visible. The medial capsule and ligament disappear from the field of view. The posterior incline of the posterior band is clearly seen. At its most posterior edge, a few fine, superficial synovial vessels may be seen extending for a short distance onto the surface of the disc. These vessels correspond to the knife-edged anterior prolongation of the synovium over the posterior incline of the posterior band (Fig. 1-26). The vessels have a transverse orientation.

MIDDLE-MEDIAL (M_m), MIDDLE-CENTRAL (M_c), AND MIDDLE-LATERAL (M_l) FIELDS

Anatomic structures readily identified in these fields include posterior incline of the posterior band, crest of the posterior band, medial capsular ligament, and synovium of the glenoid fossa.

The posterior band, like the remainder of the disc, is a uniformly smooth, stark white structure (Plate 8). Surface irregularities are unusual; when they occur, the clinician should be alerted to the possible presence of remodeled retrodiscal tissue (Plate 22). The posterior incline of the posterior band slopes obliquely against the shadow of the glenoid fossa. The mobility of the posterior band can be assessed visually by gently prodding the disc with the tip of the telescope. Similarly, the firm consistency of the posterior band may be compared with the pliable nature of the retrodiscal tissue. The joint space above the posterior incline of the posterior band is trapezoidal and oriented from posteroinferior to anterosuperior (Plate 8). The gray-white striations of the medial capsular ligament are more evident when viewed from the middle fields. The ligament is topographi-

cally related to the posterior band. Generally it is not visible in the middle-central and middle-lateral fields. Small vessels course superiorly from the medial sulcus over the surface of the capsular ligament. Pulsations of deeper vascular structures may be transmitted to the capsule.

ANTERIOR-MEDIAL (A_m), ANTERIOR-CENTRAL (A_c), AND ANTERIOR-LATERAL (A_l) FIELDS

Anatomic structures identified in these fields include anterior incline of the posterior band, medial capsule, termination of the medial capsular ligament, synovium of the glenoid fossa, and intermediate zone.

The clinician should know that the glenoid fossa tapers medially, and thus the medial fields are more apt to slightly overlap.

The anterior incline of the posterior band slopes inferiorly. As the telescope is withdrawn in a posterolateral direction, the operator appreciates the intimate relationship of the disc to the posterior slope of the eminence. The joint space above this incline is trapezoidal and oriented posterosuperiorly to anteroinferiorly. The medial capsular ligament terminates abruptly at the level of the anterior incline of the posterior band. The edge of the medial capsular ligament appears somewhat thickened. The medial capsule may continue anteriorly at a deeper plane than the ligament, because the pressure of the irrigation fluid displaces the unsupported capsule more readily than it does the ligament-supported portion of the capsule. The anterior incline blends subtly into the intermediate zone. This region cannot be recognized arthroscopically as a distinct geographic area. Again, withdrawing the telescope may increase perception of this area as the disc resumes its position of contact with the eminence and infratemporal articulating surface.

LONGITUDINAL EXAMINATION PHASE

These arthroscopic findings are described according to lateral, central, and medial fields. The longitudinal phase is a significant yet often neglected portion of the examination. The operator performs this phase primarily to confirm the presence of firm, stark white tissue—that is, the disc—in the pre-eminence region. The operator makes note of surface irregularities in the synovium and disc and the presence or absence of adhesions.

LATERAL FIELD

Anatomic structures visualized include disc, synovium lining the posterior slope of the glenoid fossa, apex of the eminence, infratemporal articulating surface of the temporal bone, lateral sulcus, and lateral capsule/ligament and anterolateral capsule. The concavity of the intermediate zone is seen to be congruent (parallel) with the convexity of the eminence (Plate 5). The presence of an anterior band can only be inferred by noting the gentle superior sloping of stark white tissue. This tissue appears to conform to the shape of the eminence. The lateral sulcus is typically distorted by the presence of the telescope as it is inserted between disc and eminence. The attachment of the lateral capsule to the eminence and disc is seen in the lateral fields.

CENTRAL FIELD

Anatomic structures visualized include disc, (intermediate zone), apex of the eminence, infratemporal articulating surface of the temporal bone, and anterior capsule. If the telescope slips posteriorly into the anterior glenoid region, the congruence of the eminence and anterior incline of the posterior band becomes obvious. The lateral capsule/ligament and medial capsule are typically not seen in this field.

MEDIAL FIELD

Anatomic structures visualized include disc, (intermediate zone), anterior capsule, and medial capsule. The interlacing fiber network of the medial capsule contrasts sharply with the strong ligamentous bands of the medial capsular ligament seen earlier in the posterior glenoid region (Plates 10 and 11). The pyramidal shape of the superior joint space is especially appreciated in the medial field. The apex of this space is located anterior and medial to its lateral boundary. The convexity of the eminence matches (parallels) the concavity of the intermediate zone of the disc. This relationship is no longer evident, once the telescope has entered the pre-eminence region.

DYNAMIC TRANSVERSE PHASE

The operator performs this portion of the examination to confirm that the condyle is lodged against the stark white tissue when the assistant distracts the mandible in an anterior and inferior direction. The tympanic portion of the retrodiscal tissue appears to alternately stretch and collapse like an accordion, when the condyle is distracted forward and backward. Still photography demonstrates this phenomenon less well than video photography.

REFERENCES

Heffez L, Blaustein DI: Diagnostic arthroscopy of the temporomandibular joint. Part 1: Normal arthroscopic findings. Oral Surg 64(6):653–678, 1987.

SUGGESTED READINGS

Blaustein DI, Heffez L: Diagnostic arthroscopy of the temporomandibular joint. Part 11: Pathological arthroscopic findings. Oral Surg 66(2):135–141, 1988.
Murakami KI, Hoshino K: Regional anatomical nomenclature and arthroscopic terminology in human temporomandibular joints. Okajimas Folia Anat Jpn 58:745–760, 1982.

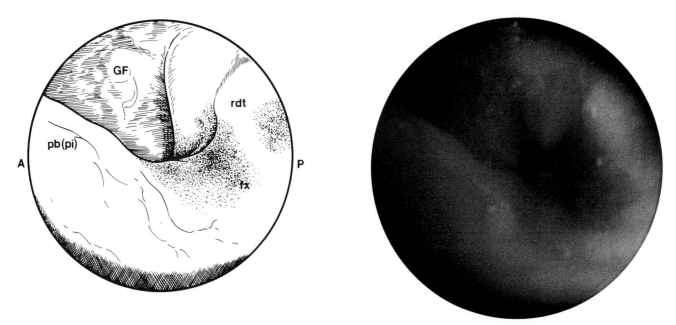

PLATE 1. Fresh Cadaver. Normal Condyle-Disc-Fossa Relationship. Left TMJ. Transverse Phase; Posterior-medial (P_m) Field.

Blood has stained the site of the flexure (fx). The fibrous connective tissue—covered glenoid fossa (GF) is in the background. No comments can be made about the superficial vascularity of the retrodiscal tissue (rdt) in the fresh cadaver specimen. The posterior attachment, stained with blood, overlies the rise of the posterior incline of the posterior band (pb (pi)). The medial sulcus is not visible here. It would lie farther medially. (**A** = anterior. **P** = posterior.)

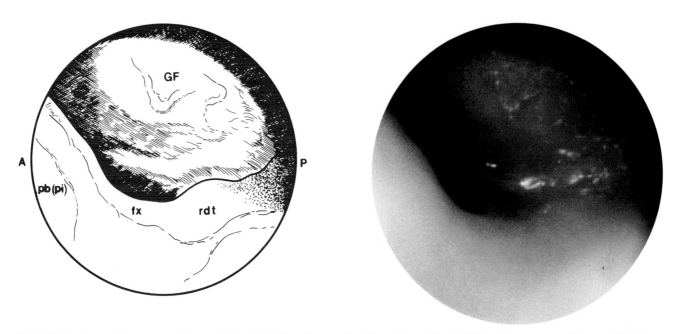

PLATE 2. Fresh Cadaver. Normal Condyle-Disc-Fossa Relationship. Right TMJ. Transverse Phase; Middle-medial (M_m) Field

The flexure (fx) has been flattened by the shaft of the telescope. Nevertheless, one can appreciate the transition in color, from pink to stark white, as one moves from the retrodiscal tissue (rdt) to the rise of the posterior incline of the posterior band (pb (pi)). The fibrous connective tissue—lined glenoid fossa (GF) is in the background. The shallow groove of the medial sulcus has been obscured by the light reflections on the synovium. (**A** = anterior. **P** = posterior.)

71

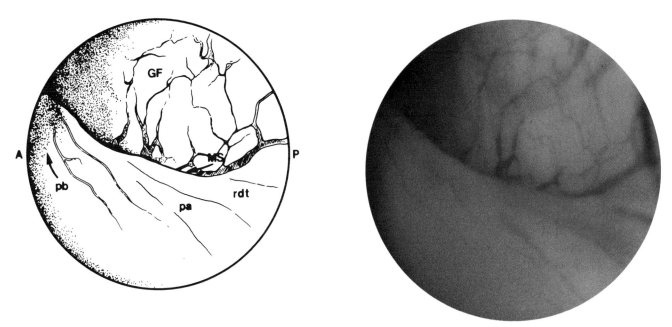

PLATE 3. Live Patient. Normal Condyle-Disc-Fossa Relationship. Left TMJ. Transverse Phase; Posterior-central (P$_c$) Field.

Retrodiscal tissue (rdt) descends obliquely in an inferior direction from the posterior aspect of the synovium-lined glenoid fossa (GF) inferiorly onto the posterior attachment (pa). Note the few transverse superficial vessels of the synovium lining the articular surface of the posterior attachment. The posterior attachment is contiguous anteriorly with the posterior incline of the posterior band (pb). This latter structure rises inferosuperiorly from posterior to anterior. The posterior limit of the medial sulcus (MS) may also be appreciated. Note that the vessels of the synovium of the glenoid fossa appear to arise from the medial sulcus, diminishing in caliber as they extend superiorly. The small demilune to the right of the field (Color Plate) resulted from a scratch on the lens of the telescope. (**A** = anterior. **P** = posterior.)

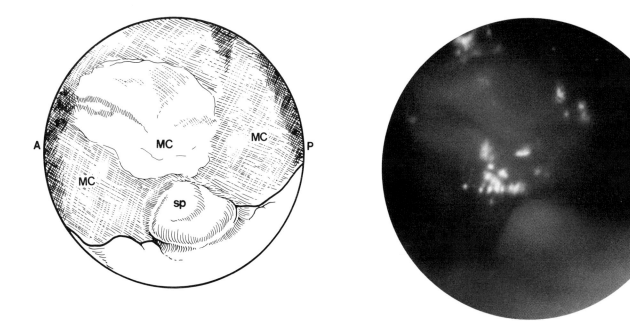

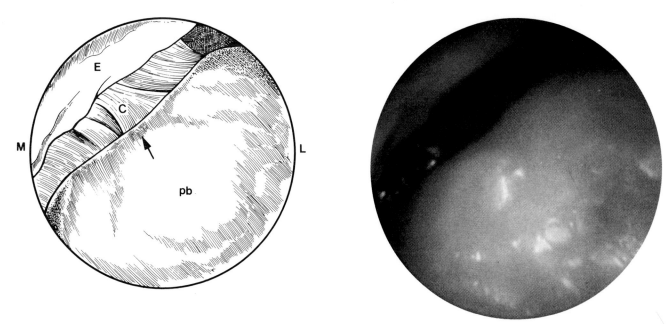

PLATE 5. Fresh Cadaver. Normal Condyle-Disc-Fossa Relationship. Right TMJ. Longitudinal Study; Medial (M) Field.

Note the fibrous connective tissue–covered eminence (E) above, and the posterior band (pb) of the disc below. The curvature of the eminence parallels that of the disc in the normal condyle-disc-fossa relationship. A groove (arrow) present on the superior surface of the disc interrupts the convex curvature of the disc. In the background, note the anterior recess of the superior joint space bounded anteriorly by the anterior capsule (C). (**M** = medial, **L** = lateral.)

PLATE 4. Fresh Cadaver. Normal Condyle-Disc-Fossa Relationship. Left TMJ. Transverse Phase; Posterior-medial (P_m) Field.

A synovial plica (sp) is noted in the most posteromedial aspect of the superior joint space. The plica is located at the reflection of the medial capsule (MC) onto the disc and retrodiscal tissues. This reflection results in the formation of a medial sulcus. Appreciation of the medial sulcus is heightened by moving the telescope gently backward and forward from medial to lateral. During normal condylar translation, the plica is stretched forward and disappears. (**A** = anterior. **P** = posterior.)

FOLLOWING PAGE

PLATES 6 to 9. Live Patient. Right TMJ

A series of four illustrations depicting decreased vascularity of the retrodiscal tissue and a superior joint space adhesion in a patient with chronic limited mouth opening following an incident of prolonged condylar dislocation. A normal condyle-disc-fossa relationship is present. In this series of illustrations, the telescope is gradually moved posteroanteriorly in the glenoid regions.

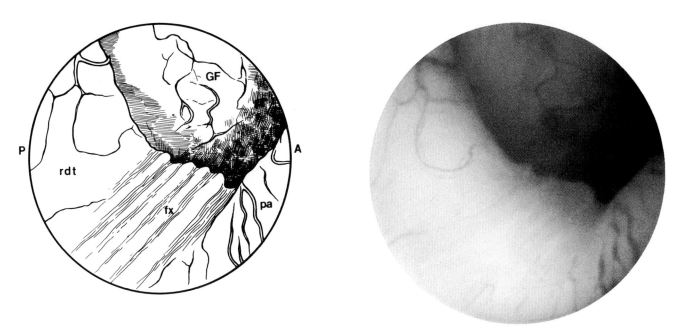

PLATE 6. Live Patient. Normal Condyle-Disc-Fossa Relationship. Right TMJ. Transverse Phase; Posterior-central (P$_c$) Field.

The flexure (fx) is in view. Note that the tympanic portion of the retrodiscal tissue (rdt) is yellow-white and has a few superficial vessels with no clear-cut orientation. In the normal disc relationship, the retrodiscal tissue displays the pink-red appearance of a highly vascular tissue. This contrasts with the transverse orientation of the few vessels noted immediately anterior to the flexure. The latter vessels belong to the posterior attachment (pa). (In Plate 7, the vessels are noted to terminate abruptly where the posterior attachment ends.) The initial rise of the posterior incline of the posterior band underlies the prolongation of the posterior attachment. The superficial vessels of the posterior attachment are visible anterior to the flexure. The retrodiscal tissue in the flexure appears white and corrugated. Superficial vessels are noticeably absent in the flexure itself. This tissue differs markedly, in both color and apparent texture, from the tympanic portion of the retrodiscal tissue. Small-caliber tortuous vessels are visible in the synovium-lined glenoid fossa (GF). (**P** = posterior. **A** = anterior.)

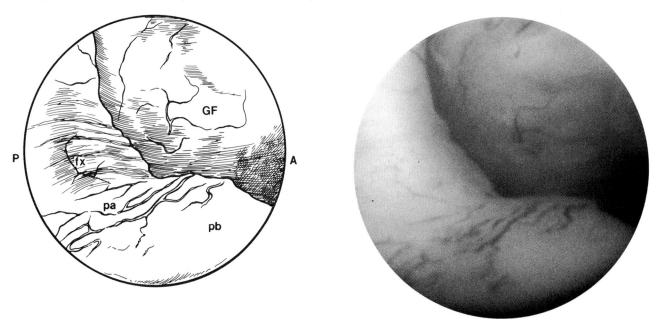

PLATE 7. Live Patient. Normal Condyle-Disc-Fossa Relationship. Right TMJ. Transverse Phase; Posterior-central (P$_c$) Field.

The morphology of the flexure (fx) has been distorted by the pressure of the telescope. The boundary between the posterior attachment (pa) and the posterior incline of the posterior band (pb) is clearly visible. Several transverse superficial vessels are seen in the posterior attachment. The synovium-lined glenoid fossa (GF) has a few vessels coursing through it. The surface of the synovium appears somewhat irregular. This finding may represent iatrogenic trauma. (**P** = posterior. **A** = anterior.)

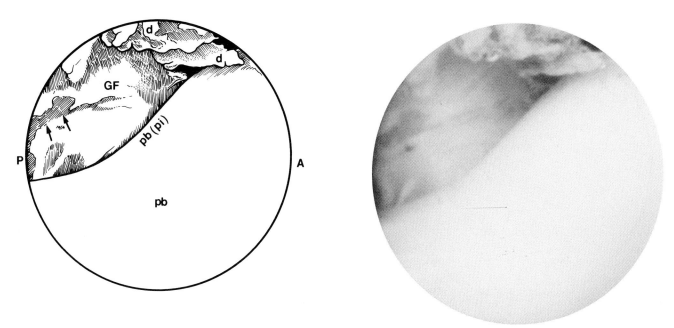

PLATE 8.   Live Patient.   Normal Condyle-Disc-Fossa Relationship.   Right TMJ.   Transverse Phase; Middle-middle (M_m) Field.

The posterior incline of the posterior band (pb (pi)) is in view. Some intra-articular debris (d) is present in the upper part of the field, partially obscuring the fibrous connective tissue–lined glenoid fossa (GF). Some of the synovium has been stripped, exposing the underlying cartilage and bony surface (arrows). Note the joint space configuration over the posterior incline of the posterior band, posteroinferior to anterosuperior. (**P** = posterior. **A** = anterior.)

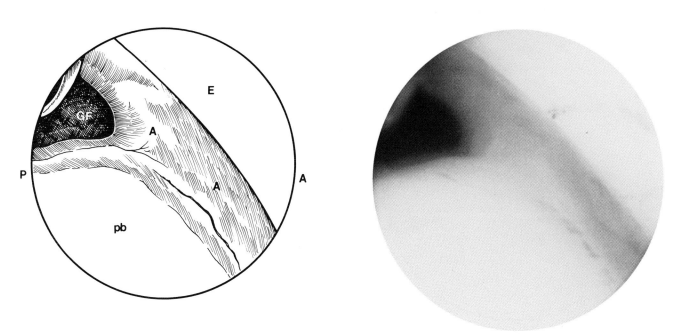

PLATE 9.   Live Patient.   Normal Condyle-Disc-Fossa Relationship.   Right TMJ.   Transverse Phase; Anterior-central (A_c) Field.

A thick, smooth band extends from the posterior slope of the eminence (E) to the anterior incline of the posterior band (pb), encroaching on its crest. The band represents an adhesion (A). In this particular case, the stark white color of the posterior band does not differ markedly from that of the fibrous connective tissue–covered eminence. In contrast, the adhesion has a distinctive yellow color. The glenoid fossa (GF) is in the dark background and is not visible. (**P** = posterior. **A** = anterior.)

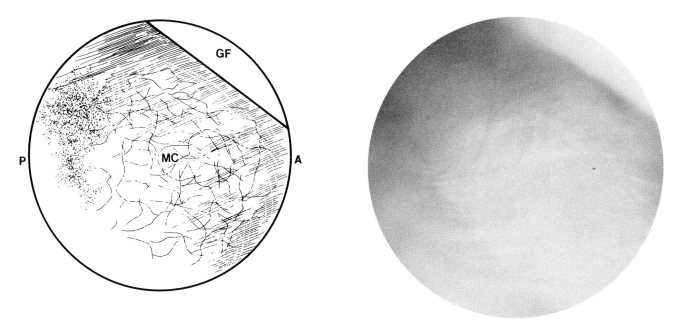

PLATE 10. Live Patient. Normal Condyle-Disc-Fossa Relationship. Right TMJ. Transverse Examination Phase.

The telescope is positioned to inspect the medial capsule (MC). Note its delicate interlacing fibers. Compare this fiber arrangement to that seen in the medial capsular ligament (Plate 11). To the left of the field the tissue appears stained with blood. No superficial synovial vessels are present. The ivory-colored glenoid fossa (GF) is seen to the right of the field. (**P** = posterior. **A** = anterior.)

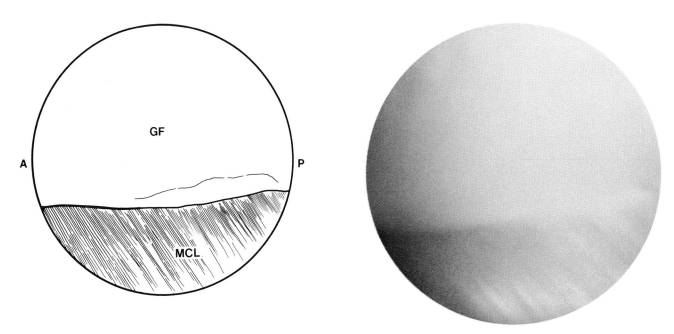

PLATE 11. Live Patient. Normal Condyle-Disc-Fossa Relationship. Left TMJ. Transverse Phase.

The telescope is positioned to inspect the attachment of the medial capsular ligament (MCL) to the glenoid fossa (GF). No joint space is appreciated. No superficial vessels are visible. The posteroinferior to anterosuperior orientation of the fibers should be noted. The gray-blue color of the ligament contrasts with the ivory color of the fibrous connective tissue–lined glenoid fossa. (**A** = anterior. **P** = posterior.)

PATHOLOGIC ARTHROSCOPIC ANATOMY

6

This chapter discusses the arthroscopic pathologic conditions associated with internal derangements of the temporomandibular joint. The criteria for disc displacements were established by correlating clinical and imaging findings with complete arthroscopic examinations of the superior joint space. Images used in the assessment of the disc-fossa relationship consisted of sagittal horizontally and vertically corrected cephalometric arthrotomograms, uncorrected sagittal and coronal double-contrast computed tomograms, or uncorrected sagittal and coronal magnetic resonance images (Rosenberg, Graczyk, 1986, Heffez et al., 1988).

As in Chapter 5, the text is referenced with plates selected from those at the end of the chapter.

A spectrum of changes has been noted, arthroscopically, in the internally deranged joint. The clinician must learn to describe color, surface morphology, texture, orientation of structures, joint space configuration, and topographic relationships for each field of vision examined. In this mannner, the clinician learns to piece together a composite picture of the diagnostic problem.

An anatomic nomenclature was created to describe structures or features absent from the normal arthroscopic examination. The nomenclature is reviewed below.

An *adhesion* is a fibrous connective tissue band fixed at both ends. Adhesions may be further defined using the descriptors *linear* (Plate 34) or *weblike* (Plate 9).

Corrugations are small, surface foldings within a tissue. They are especially apparent in the remodeled retrodiscal tissue at the site of the flexure, where the tissue appears compressed like an accordion (Plate 19).

The term *depression* is used to describe an interruption in the normal topography of a structure. A depression in the medial capsular ligament may occur iatrogenically if the trocar is directed too far medially (Plate 53).

A structure is described as **fibrillated** when the surface is composed of fibrils. This term is often used to describe extremely remodeled retrodiscal tissue (Plate 22).

A *fold (pleat)* refers to a thickened cordlike structure within the tympanic portion of the retrodiscal tissue. Typically a medial fold and lateral fold are present (Plates 14 to 16)

The term *remodeled posterior band* or *remodeled disc* is used to describe the altered shape and thus the altered internal fiber architecture of the disc. The term is used as a descriptor in arthroscopy and imaging. Disc remodeling may be confirmed arthroscopically by noting the flattening of the posterior band in the superior joint space. This flattening accommodates the eminence and infratemporal articulating surface of the temporal bone. Disc remodeling is responsible for the change in configuration of the superior joint space.

Remodeled retrodiscal tissue (remodeled posterior attachment) represents tissue originating from the posterior attachment that has been progressively pulled over the condyle as the disc is displaced anteromedially. The tissue displays a variable degree of superficial vascularity, presumably as a result of differential loading.

Transverse, longitudinal, and dynamic examination phases are performed and arthroscopic findings recorded and described according to fields of view

(Chapter 5). The arthroscopic findings of the internally deranged joint are described according to the phase of the examination in which they are observed (Heffez, Blaustein, 1987, Blaustein, Heffez, 1988)

TRANSVERSE EXAMINATION PHASE

In the transverse examination phase, the diagnosis of anterior disc displacement is supported by the finding of dull white or ivory-colored tympanic retrodiscal tissue; the presence of tissue with varying degrees of superficial vascularity in the glenoid region; a funnel-shaped superior joint space; fibrillation of tissue surfaces; and the presence of tissue with transverse vascularity at the level of the termination of the medial capsular ligament.

The *flexure* in the internally deranged joint is formed by the junction of the retrodiscal tissue originating from the tympanic plate and the remodeled retrodiscal tissue now draped over the condylar head (Plate 17). The tympanic portion of the retrodiscal tissue loses its pink color and becomes dull white or ivory. Compare the color of this structure in the slight disc displacement (Plate 12) with that found in the chronic disc displacement (Plate 24).

The anterior positioning of the posterior band results in a change in the configuration of the superior joint space. In the normal disc relationship, the space is oriented posteroinferiorly to anterosuperiorly in the posterior glenoid regions. In more practical terms, the telescope must travel inferosuperiorly to reach the anterior glenoid region in the normal relationship. In the displaced disc, minimal movement of the telescope is required to complete a sweep of the glenoid region. The flexure may be more easily distorted by the pressure of the telescope and by the dilation of the space, because the remodeled retrodiscal tissue is softer and more pliable than the disc. As a result, the flexure is more sharply defined, forming a V rather than a U, as in the normal condyle-disc-fossa relationship. The presence of remodeled retrodiscal tissue is the hallmark of the internally deranged joint.

The tissue is most readily identified in the transverse examination phase by locating superficial transverse vessels. The degrees and patterns of this vascularity vary (Plates 20 and 29). As one proceeds with the examination in a posteroanterior direction, several distinct zones of vascularity may be identified. The zones in any one field of view are typically numbered alphanumerically from posterior to anterior, by attaching a subscript to the capital letter Z (for example, Zone 1 is Z_1). Alternatively, the remodeled retrodiscal tissue may be described as load-bearing or nonload-bearing, depending on the findings of the dynamic examination phase. During this phase, the condyle will appear to load areas that demonstrate poor or absent vascularity. The zones of vascularity are not always evident, especially when significant tissue remodeling has occurred (Plate 26). Under these circumstances, the clinician may mistake remodeled retrodiscal tissue for disc. The prudent clinician looks for color similarities between the coverings of the eminence/glenoid fossa and the covering of the unknown structure. When the color of the structure below approaches the yellow-white or gray-white color of the eminence/glenoid fossa, one should suspect remodeled retrodiscal tissue. No other structure seen in the superior joint space has the stark white color of the disc. In addition, close inspection of the surface may reveal surface irregularities as well as fibrillations (Plate 22). As remodeling proceeds, the lateral fields of view show greater signs of remodeling than the medial. This finding agrees with the conclusions of Hansson and Oberg (1976), who found greater arthrotic and morphologic changes in the lateral third of the condyles examined.

Occasionally, only a patch of superficial vessels barely filling one field of view is noted on an ivory-colored tissue (Plate 35). The tissue resembles the pannus of rheumatoid arthritis. The term pannus should not be used for this condition, however, as the pannus is a membrane covering a *normal* surface (Stedman's, 1982).

In the normal disc relationship, the synovium overlying the posterior attachment never exists farther anteriorly than the posterior incline of the posterior band (Fig. 1-26). On arthroscopic examination, the junction between the posterior attachment and the remodeled posterior band is well demarcated (Plate 21). It is readily identified by the abrupt termination of the few superficial transverse vessels of the posterior attachment and the stark whiteness of the posterior incline of the posterior band. The vessels of the posterior attachment overlying the posterior band do not always have an obvious transverse orientation and typically are few. The presence of superficial vascularity in and beyond the middle fields likely indicates the presence of an internally deranged joint.

The medial capsular ligament has been discussed previously as an important topographic landmark. The fibers appear gray-white and are typically oriented in a posteroinferior to anterosuperior direction when the condyle is depressed and only slightly forward (Plate 18). This is the standard condylar position when the examination is performed without active joint distraction. The anterior extent of the ligament is obvious on examination. In the normal condyle-disc-fossa relationship, the ligament's abrupt termination should correspond with the stark white posterior band. When this landmark is related to vascular tissue, the operator should strongly suspect the presence of remodeled retrodiscal tissue and thus an anterior disc displacement (Plate 18). The medial capsular ligament should not be confused with an adhesion.

Occasionally, perforations of the remodeled retrodiscal tissue have been observed (Plate 39). The perforations have typically been seen in the lateral and central fields during the transverse examination phase. They have never been observed in the pre-eminence region. The remodeled retrodiscal tissue surrounding the perforations has little superficial vascularity and is dull white to ivory (Plates 39 and 41). No perforations have been observed in areas of high superficial vascularity. Air insufflation of the superior joint space may facilitate localization of the perforations, by virtue of an increase in the field of vision and greater compression of the retrodiscal tissue against the condyle during function.

Medial and lateral folds (pleats) have been noted in the tympanic portion of the retrodiscal tissue of the internally deranged joint (Plate 16). The prominence of these structures in the internally deranged joint may be important. One should be cautious in assigning any major significance to this finding at this time, however, because far more live human internally deranged joints than normal joints have been examined arthroscopically.

LONGITUDINAL EXAMINATION PHASE

In the longitudinal examination phase, the arthroscopist looks for the lack of congruity or parallelism between the silhouette of the remodeled retrodiscal tissue and the covering of the eminence. In addition, the remodeled retrodiscal tissue may be seen to extend anteriorly, where it abruptly meets and is contiguous with the stark white disc. This junction is most obvious when a high concentration of blood vessels is present in the remodeled retrodiscal tissue. Increasing degrees of remodeling, inferred from the decrease in the number of superficial vessels, may make identification of the junction difficult. With extreme remodeling the operator relies mostly on color to indicate where the disc begins. Fibrillations and surface irregularities may also guide the operator (Plate 36).

The mismatching or lack of parallelism between the remodeled retrodiscal tissue and the fibrous connective tissue–covered eminence is evident during this phase of the examination (Plate 27). An hourglass

configuration is formed between these tissues. In the normal condyle-disc-eminence relationship, the disc maintains contact with the eminence, as the telescope more readily displaces remodeled retrodiscal tissue than disc. Arthroscopically this is inferred from the matching of the curvature of the disc (intermediate zone) with that of the eminence. Noting this change is particularly helpful when the retrodiscal tissue is heavily remodeled.

DYNAMIC TRANSVERSE PHASE

During the dynamic transverse phase, the superficial vessels appear to empty during opening and fill during closing. This apparent paradox may occur because of internal rerouting of blood to the deeper venous plexuses as the retrodiscal tissue is stretched. It may also be due to the presence of irrigation fluid and the manipulation of the telescope. It is not possible to assess disc reduction using superior joint space arthroscopy.

When a perforation of the remodeled retrodiscal tissue is located, the head of the condyle may be seen protruding through it. Under these circumstances, the fibrous connective tissue covering of the condyle has not always appeared intact (Plate 39). Whether this represents a pathologic condition or the result of iatrogenia cannot be definitively stated. Occasionally, granulation tissue appears to have protruded from the inferior joint space (Plate 41).

The articular cartilaginous surfaces of the temporal bone and condyle are covered with a fibrous connective tissue (Chapter 2). In our experience, unlike in arthroscopy of the osteoarthrotic knee (Altman, Gray, 1983), ulcerations, yellowing, softening of cartilage, and exposure of osseous surfaces cannot be evaluated, at least in the early and usually asymptomatic phase of the disease.

The fibrous connective tissues covering the glenoid fossa and eminence generally appear intact in the presence of advanced remodeling of the retrodiscal tissue. Several authors have used *articular fibrillation* (Hellsing et al., 1984, Sanders, 1986) to describe the fraying of synovium. In our experience, much of the fraying of synovium and subsequent denudation of the glenoid fossa/eminence is secondary to iatrogenia from the trocar or telescope. A greater amount of floating debris is noted with the duration of the examination and repeated entries.

Adhesions have not been commonly noted in disc displacements. Small weblike bands have been observed along the medial sulcus in posteromedial fields and in the pre-eminence region where the anterior attachment joins with the capsule. These adhesions span a short distance. Linear bands have been observed extending from the posterior slope of the eminence to the disc or remodeled retrodiscal tissue (Plate 34). These adhesions are more conspicuous than the weblike bands. Adhesions may occur in the normal condyle-disc-fossa relationships (Plate 9).

DIAGNOSTIC MARKERS FOR DISC DISPLACEMENT

1. The tympanic portion of the retrodiscal tissue loses its pink color and becomes dull white or ivory.

2. A flexure composed of the junction of the tympanic portion of retrodiscal tissue with remodeled retrodiscal tissue is identified.

3. Remodeled retrodiscal tissue is seen in the glenoid regions. This tissue is remarkable for the presence of superficial vascularity. The vessels course through a tissue that is dull, yellow-white, or ivory.

4. Tissue with superficial vascularity is present at the level of the termination of the medial capsular ligament.

5. A perforation is present.

6. A funnel-shaped joint space is identified in the posterior fields, with the firm disc being displaced anteriorly.

7. Tissue fibrillations and surface irregularities are noted.

8. In the longitudinal examination phase, the convexity of the remodeled retrodiscal tissue does not match (lack of congruence) the convexity of the eminence, resulting in an hourglass configuration.

9. In the dynamic examination phase, the condyle appears to contact remodeled retrodiscal tissue (a yellow-white structure bearing transverse superficial vascularity) and not the disc (a stark white, glistening avascular structure).

These diagnostic markers will be used in the text descriptions associated with the arthroscopic illustrations.

REFERENCES

Altman RD, Gray R: Diagnostic and therapeutic uses of the arthroscope in rheumatoid arthritis and osteoarthritis. Am J Med 75(4B):50–55, 1983.

Blaustein DI, Heffez L: Diagnostic arthroscopy of the temporomandibular joint. Part 11: Pathological arthroscopic findings. Oral Surg 66(2):135–141, 1988.

Hansson T, Oberg T: Arthrosis and deviation in form in the temporomandibular joint. A macroscopic study on a human autopsy material. Acta Odont Scand 35:167–174, 1976.

Heffez L, Blaustein DI: Diagnostic arthrosocopy of the temporomandibular joint. Part 1: Normal arthroscopic findings. Oral Surg 64(6):653–678, 1987.

Heffez L, Mafee MF, Langer B, et al. Double contrast arthrography of the temporomandibular joint: Role of direct sagittal CT imaging. Oral Surg 65:511–514, 1988.

Hellsing G, Holmlund A, Nordenram A, et al. Arthroscopy of the temporomandibular joint. Examination of two patients with suspected disk derangement. Int J Oral Surg 13:69–74, 1984.

Rosenberg HM, Graczyk RJ: Temporomandibular articulation tomography: a corrected anteroposterior and lateral cephalometric technique. Oral Surg 62:198, 1986.

Sanders B, Buoncristiani R: Diagnostic and surgical arthroscopy of the temporomandibular joint. Clinical experience with 137 procedures over a two year period. J Craniomand Pract 1:202–213, 1987.

Stedman's Medical Dictionary, 24th ed, Baltimore Williams & Wilkins, 1982.

SUGGESTED READINGS

Eriksson L, Westesson PL: Deterioration of temporary silicone implant in the temporomandibular joint. A clinical and arthroscopic follow-up study. Oral Surg 62:2–6, 1986.

Holmlund A, Hellsing G:Arthroscopy of the temporomandibular joint. An autopsy study. Int J Oral surg 14:169–75, 1985.

Murakami K, Hoshino K: Regional anatomical nomenclature and arthroscopic terminology in human tempormandibular joints. Okajimas Folla Anat Jpn 58:745–760, 1982.

Murakami K, Matsuki M, Iizuka T, et al. Diagnostic arthroscopy of the TMJ: Differential diagnoses in patients with limited jaw opening. J Craniomand Pract 4:117–126, 1986.

Nuelle D, Alpern MC and Ufema JW: Arthroscopic surgery of the temporomandibular joint. The Angle Orthodontist 56:118–141, 1986.

Sanders B: Arthroscopic surgery of tempormandibular joint: Treatment of internal derangement with persistent closed lock. Oral Surg 62:361–372, 1986.

PLATE 13.   Disc Displacement With Reduction.   Left TMJ.   Transverse Phase; Posterior-medial (P$_m$) Field.

The flexure (arrow) is in view. The morphology of this flexure may be due to several factors, including the position of the telescope and the fluid dilation of the joint space. The flexure represents the junction of the tympanic portion of the retrodiscal tissue (rdt) and remodeled retrodiscal tissue (*rdt'*). The retrodiscal tissue appears less compact than the remodeled retrodiscal tissue. Note that the vessels of the retrodiscal tissue are not oriented transversely. This contrasts sharply with the orientation of those vessels found within the remodeled tissue. Both tissues are yellow-white. The fibrous connective tissue–lined glenoid fossa (GF) is seen in the background. (**A** = anterior. **P** = posterior.)

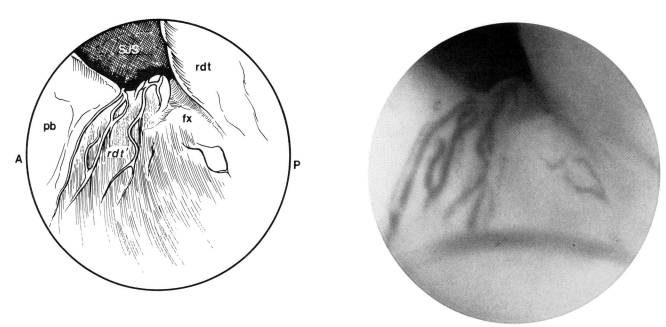

PLATE 12.   Very Slight Disc Displacement With Reduction.   Left TMJ.   Transverse Phase; Posterior-central (P$_c$) Field.

The flexure (fx) is composed of vertically oriented and horizontally oriented portions. The vertical portion represents normal pink-red retrodiscal tissue (rdt). The more lateral the telescope is positioned, the more vertical the orientation of the retrodiscal tissue. The horizontal portion represents remodeling of retrodiscal tissue (*rdt'*). Note the group of transversely oriented vessels at the junction of this tissue with the posterior incline of the posterior band (pb). A few superficial vessels are noted on the normal retrodiscal tissue. The stark white color of the posterior band contrasts sharply with the color of the retrodiscal tissues. Small-caliber synovial vessels are occasionally noted in the posterior attachment overlying the posterior band in the slight anterior disc displacement or in the normal condyle-disc-fossa relationship. The posterior incline of the posterior band appears to be rising in a posterosuperior to anterosuperior direction. The superior joint space (SJS) is noted. (**A** = anterior. **P** = posterior.)

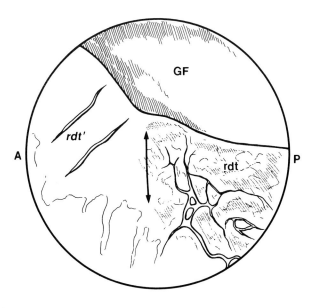

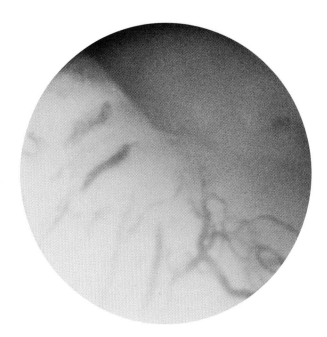

PLATE 13.   See opposite page for legend.

PLATES 14 to 16. Disc Displacement With Reduction. Right TMJ. Transverse Phase; Posterior-central (P_c) Field.

A series of illustrations demonstrating how the tympanic portion of the retrodiscal tissue relates to the fibrous connective tissue–lined glenoid fossa. In this series, several views of the same POSTERIOR-central (P_c) field have been obtained. The flexure can be exaggerated by the presence of the telescope and dilation by the irrigation fluid. See specific plate descriptions, below.

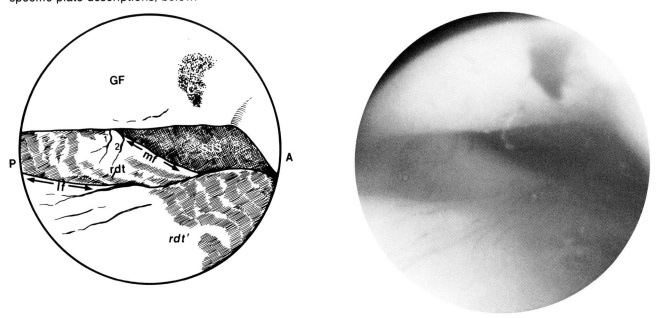

PLATE 14

The transversely oriented vessels (1,2) of the retrodiscal tissue (rdt) appear small in caliber. The distracting glare from the light on the fibrous connective tissue–lined glenoid fossa (GF) makes comparing its color and vascular patterns with those of the retrodiscal tissue difficult. A depression in the retrodiscal tissue is flanked by two elevations, medial fold (mf) and lateral fold (lf). The depression appears to match the topography of this glenoid fossa. Immediately anterior to the retrodiscal tissue lies the remodeled retrodiscal tissue (*rdt'*). Superiorly, there is a small blood clot (c) on the glenoid fossa. (**P** = posterior. **A** = anterior.)

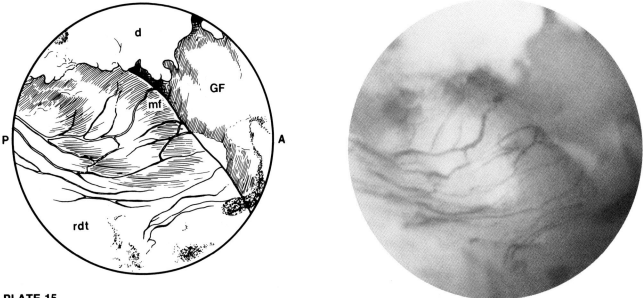

PLATE 15

The valley in the tympanic portion of the retrodiscal tissue (rdt) is closely inspected. The medial fold (mf) is in view. Fine transversely oriented vessels are noted. These are the same vessels as labeled in Plate 14. They appear larger in caliber because the telescope is positioned within the valley. Some debris (d) is visible in the superior aspect of the field. The debris may represent extracapsular tissue introduced iatrogenically. The fibrous connective tissue–lined glenoid fossa (GF) is in the background. (**P** = posterior. **A** = anterior.)

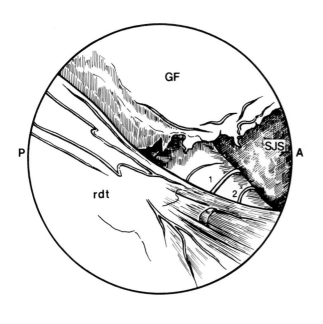

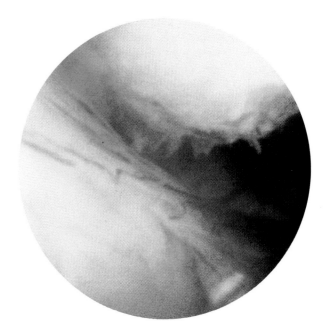

PLATE 16

Note the apparent intimate relationship of the glenoid fossa (GF) with the valley in the retrodiscal tissue (rdt). Manipulation of the telescope has caused some fraying of the synovium lining the glenoid fossa. The vessels labeled as 1 and 2 are those that appear in Plate 14. The superior joint space (SJS) is seen to the right of the field. (**P** = posterior. **A** = anterior.)

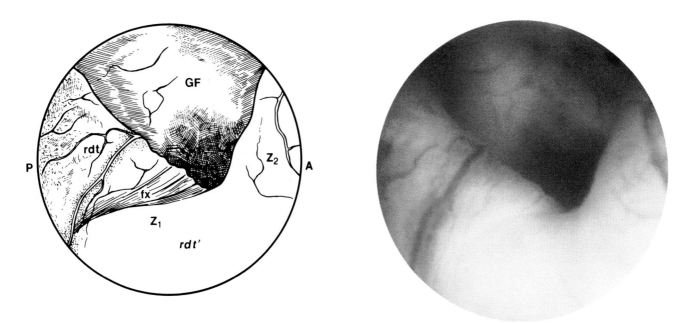

PLATE 17.   Disc Displacement With Reduction.   Right TMJ.   Transverse Phase; Posterior-central (P_c) Field.

The flexure (fx) is in view. The tissue here is distinctively white and corrugated. In the dynamic transverse phase, this tissue was noted to stretch, eliminating the corrugations. Note the remodeled retrodiscal tissue (*rdt'*) and the tympanic portion of the retrodiscal tissue (rdt). The firm, relatively smooth retrodiscal tissue contrasts with the irregular surface of the remodeled retrodiscal tissue. Transversely oriented vessels are noted on both structures. Note the two zones of relative superficial vascularity in the remodeled retrodiscal tissue. Zone 1 (Z_1) is relatively avascular, and Zone 2 (Z_2) shows prominent superficial vascularity. The synovium-lined glenoid fossa (GF) is in the background. (**P** = posterior. **A** = anterior.)

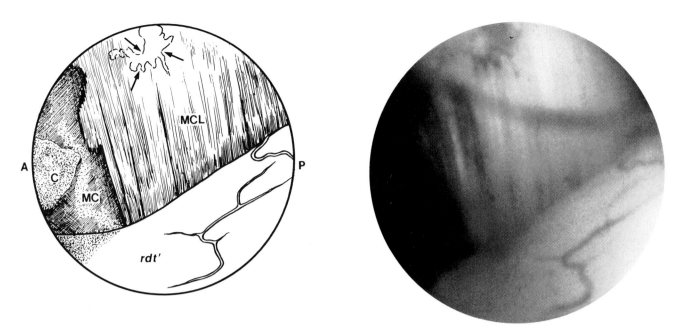

PLATE 18.   Disc Displacement With Reduction.   Left TMJ.   Transverse Phase; Middle-central (M$_c$) Field.

The obliquely oriented fibers of the medial capsular ligament (MCL) are in full view. The termination of this ligament is an important arthroscopic landmark for locating the anterior surface of the condyle. The unsupported medial capsule (MC) is noted immediately anterior to the ligament. A clot (c) lies on the capsule to the extreme left of the field. Small dilated, perhaps traumatized synovial vessels (arrows) are noted coursing on the ligament. Remodeled retrodiscal tissue (*rdt'*) is ivory colored and has a few superficial vessels oriented in a generally transverse direction. A gray demilune, visible in the Color Plate, crosses the upper half of the field. The demilune probably represents a scratch on the lens of the telescope. Had the demilune resulted from an air bubble, the image above the demilune would have been distorted, but sharper. (**A** = anterior. **P** = posterior.)

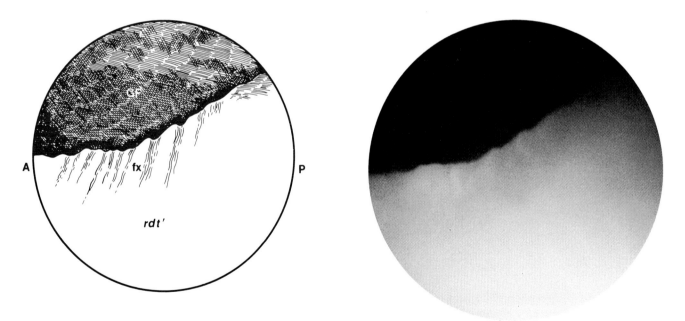

PLATE 19.   Disc Displacement With Reduction.   Left TMJ.   Dynamic Transverse Phase; Middle-central (M$_c$) Field.

The corrugated appearance of the remodeled retrodiscal tissue (*rdt'*) is obvious at the flexure (fx). The mandible has been distracted slightly forward. With further anterior distraction the corrugations would disappear. Note the absence of superficial transverse vessels. The bulk of the remodeled retrodiscal tissue appears, characteristically, yellow-white. The superior margin, where the corrugations are located, appears almost translucent, possibly due to transillumination. The glenoid fossa (GF), obscured by shadow, is barely visible. (**A** = anterior. **P** = posterior.)

84

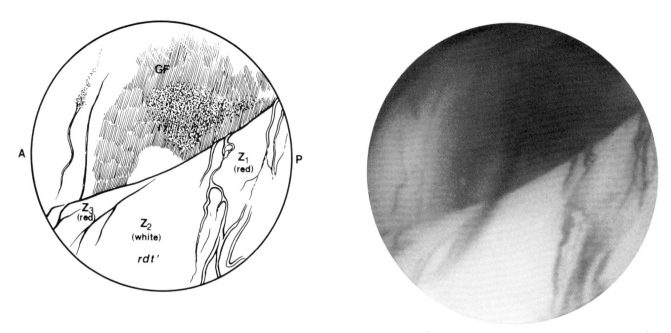

PLATE 20. Disc Displacement With Reduction. Left TMJ. Transverse Phase; Anterior-central (A_c) Field.

Three zones are present on the superficial aspect of the remodeled retrodiscal tissue (*rdt'*). The zones may be indicated by color (red, white, red) or numerically (posteroanteriorly as Z_1, Z_2, and Z_3). The zones are not always as clearly identifiable as in this plate. The transverse orientation of the vessels, however, is distinctive in the glenoid regions. Zone 2 (Z_2) of the remodeled retrodiscal tissue probably represents an area of loading. The color of this area more closely approximates the stark white color in the posterior band, not visible here. The operator could mistake Zone 2 for remodeled posterior band if the transverse examination phase is not completed. The presence of two vascular zones separated by an avascular zone is a criterion for anterior disc displacement. Note the glenoid fossa (GF) in the background. (**A** = anterior. **P** = posterior.)

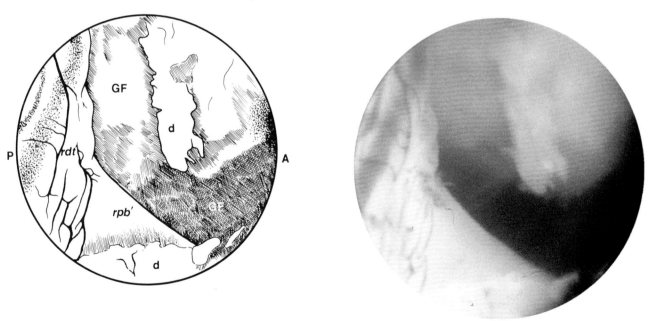

PLATE 21. Disc Displacement With Reduction. Right TMJ. Transverse Phase; Anterior-lateral (A_l) Field.

The abrupt termination of the remodeled retrodiscal tissue (*rdt'*) is observed where the transversely oriented vessels end. The operator can mentally draw a precise line representing the junction of the remodeled retrodiscal tissue with the remodeled posterior band (*rpb'*). Note the fibrous connective tissue–lined glenoid fossa (GF). Some white debris (d) partially obscures the inferior and superior aspect of the field. This tissue may represent iatrogenically introduced extracapsular tissue. The rise of the posterior incline of the posterior band is absent here, and hence the term remodeled posterior band. Without the benefit of the findings of the longitudinal examination phase, the operator could mistake this white area for an avascular zone of loaded remodeled retrodiscal tissue. The color of the remodeled posterior band is uniformly stark white, as compared to the ivory color of the glenoid fossa. (**P** = posterior. **A** = anterior.)

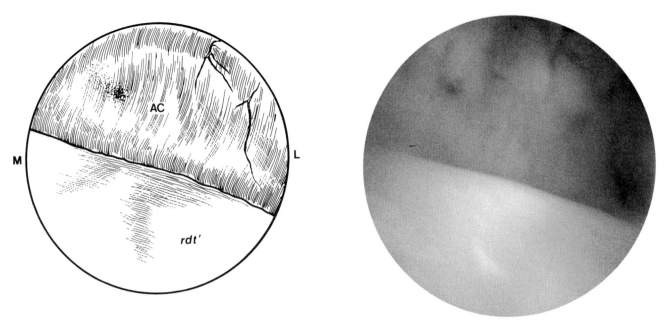

PLATE 22. Disc Displacement With Reduction. Right TMJ. Longitudinal Phase; Middle (M) Field.

The telescope is positioned in the pre-eminence region. The anterior capsule (AC) is in the background and the ivory-colored remodeled retrodiscal tissue (*rdt'*) is seen below. The capsule is formed of synovium-lined fibrous connective tissue and appears gray-blue. A few delicate synovial vessels course across the capsule. The extreme remodeling of the retrodiscal tissue is obvious when the surface is closely inspected. Compare the white and yellow areas of fibrous connective tissue to the firm-textured, smooth, stark white disc seen in Plate 11. No superficial vessels are noted in this remodeled retrodiscal tissue. (**M** = medial. **L** = lateral.)

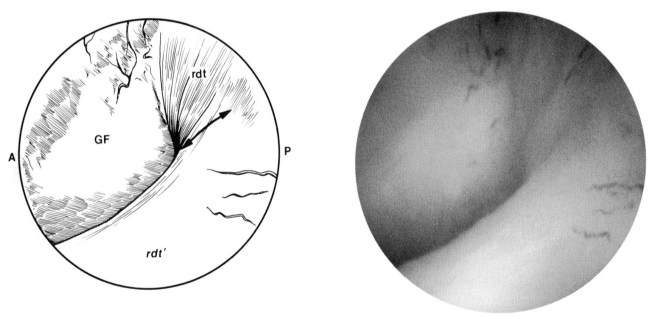

PLATE 23. Disc Displacement Without Reduction. Left TMJ. Transverse Phase; Posterior-medial (P_m) Field.

A small area of the tympanic portion of the retrodiscal tissue (rdt) is in view. Three transversely oriented superficial vessels are noted in the remodeled retrodiscal tissue (*rdt'*). These vessels are small in caliber. The most superior part of the retrodiscal tissue, where it approximates the glenoid fossa (GF), appears loose. Immediately anterior to the retrodiscal tissue is the remodeled retrodiscal tissue separated artificially by the flexure (arrows). The fibrous nature of the remodeled retrodiscal tissue is apparent on close scrutiny. The character and yellow-white color of this tissue is typical of extreme remodeling. The flexure is broad and not as accentuated as in more central and lateral fields. (**A** = anterior. **P** = posterior.)

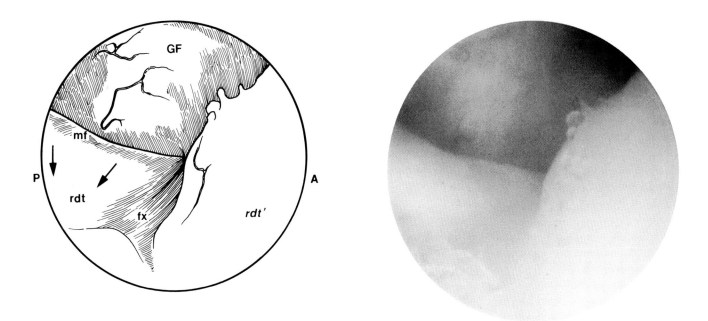

PLATE 24. Disc Displacement Without Reduction. Right TMJ. Transverse Phase; Posterior-central (P$_c$) Field.

The flexure (fx) is in view. There is minimal color difference between the tympanic portion of the retrodiscal tissue (rdt) and the remodeled retrodiscal tissue (*rdt'*). There are subtle irregularities on the surface of the remodeled retrodiscal tissue, and a small-caliber superficial vessel is present. No vessels are noted in the retrodiscal tissue. In the background are a few small-caliber vessels within the synovium of the glenoid fossa (GF). The valley (arrows) and medial fold (mf) within the retrodiscal tissue can be seen immediately posterior to the flexure. (**P** = posterior. **A** = anterior.)

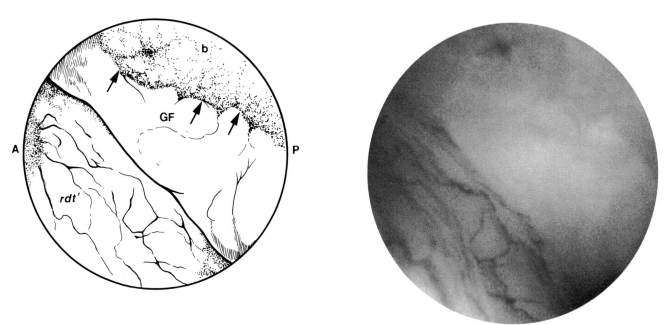

PLATE 25. Disc Displacement Without Reduction. Left TMJ. Transverse Phase; Middle-central (M$_c$) Field.

Note the remodeled retrodiscal tissue (*rdt'*) demonstrating a moderate number of superficial vessels. The vessels do not have any clear-cut transverse orientation. The texture of the tissue may be described as loose, contrasting sharply with the compact fibrous nature of extremely remodeled retrodiscal tissue (see Plate 24). The synovium of the glenoid fossa (GF) is torn (arrows), possibly due to iatrogenic scraping with the telescope or trocar. The underlying bone (b) is exposed. (**A** = anterior. **P** = posterior.)

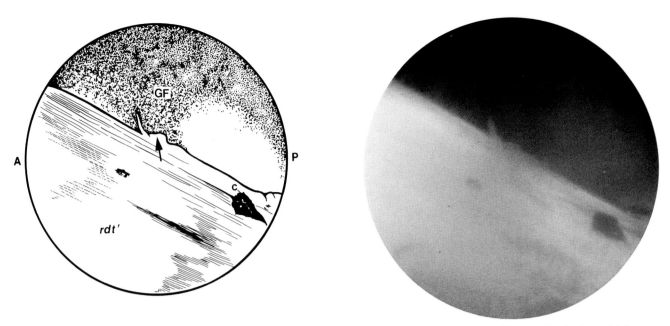

PLATE 26. Disc Displacement Without Reduction. Left TMJ. Dynamic Transverse Phase; Posterior-middle (Pₘ) Field.

The mandible has been moved forward by the assistant. The stretched, fibrous remodeled retrodiscal tissue (*rdt'*) is oriented obliquely inferosuperiorly. This structure has areas of varying texture and color. A hint of longitudinal striation is apparent within the tissue, giving the appearance of a compact fibrous connective tissue. The superior surface of this structure is irregular (arrow) and may be described as fibrillated. This feature contrasts sharply with the smooth, regular surface of the stark white disc (see Plate 8). A small clot (c) lies to the extreme right of the field. The remodeled retrodiscal tissue lacks obvious superficial vascularity. The fibrous connective tissue lining the glenoid fossa (GF) is seen in the background. The superior joint space is free of debris. (**A** = anterior. **P** = posterior.)

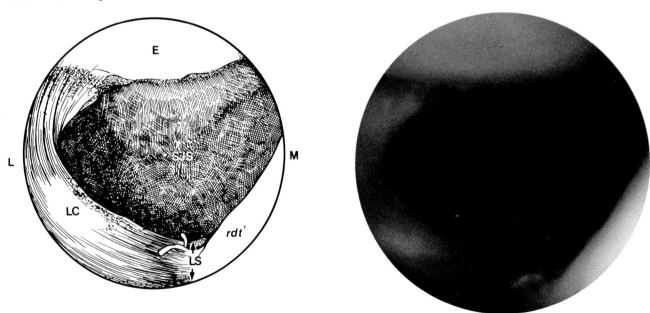

PLATE 27. Disc Displacement Without Reduction. Left TMJ. Longitudinal Phase; Lateral (L) Field.

The lateral pre-eminence region is in view. Typically, this region is limited anteriorly by the attachment of the lateral capsule (LC) and lateral ligament, restricting the examination of structures and relationships. The lateral capsule attaches to the remodeled retrodiscal tissue (*rdt'*) below and the eminence (E) above. The gray color of the lateral capsule contrasts sharply with the yellow-white color of the remodeled retrodiscal tissue and connective tissue–covered eminence. The reflection of the capsule onto the remodeled retrodiscal tissue forms the lateral sulcus (LS). The morphology of the lateral sulcus has been flattened by the telescope and by dilation with the irrigation fluid. The attachment of the lateral sulcus to the eminence is stained with blood. Note the lack of parallelism between the surface of the remodeled retrodiscal tissue and that of the eminence. The configuration of the superior joint space (SJS) is altered. There are no surface vessels in the remodeled retrodiscal tissue, eminence, or synovium covering the capsule. The anterior recess is free of debris. The remodeled disc would lie anteromedially. (**L** = lateral. **M** = medial.)

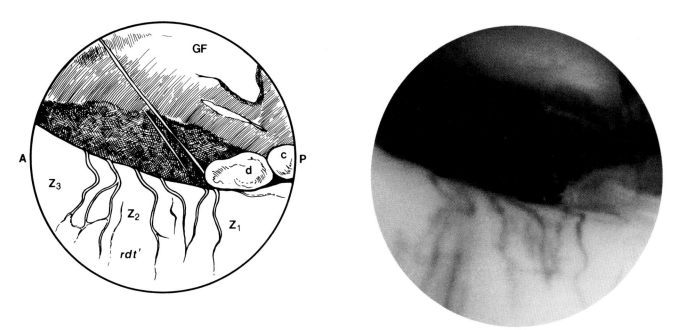

PLATE 28. Disc Displacement Without Reduction.   Left TMJ.   Transverse Phase; Middle-central (M_c)Field.

Three distinct zones are visible in the remodeled retrodiscal tissue (*rdt'*). They may be distinguished by the number of superficial vessels present in each. The zones are numbered posteroanteriorly. Zone 1 (Z_1) and Zone 3 (Z_3) have no superficial vessels. In Zone 2 (Z_2) a moderate number of superficial vessels are seen, oriented transversely. Clot (c) and debris (d) are noted posteriorly. Strands of hyaluronate-protein complex (mucin) extend from the glenoid fossa (GF) to the remodeled retrodiscal tissue. Note, above, the smooth synovial lining of the glenoid fossa. (**A** = anterior. **P** = posterior.)

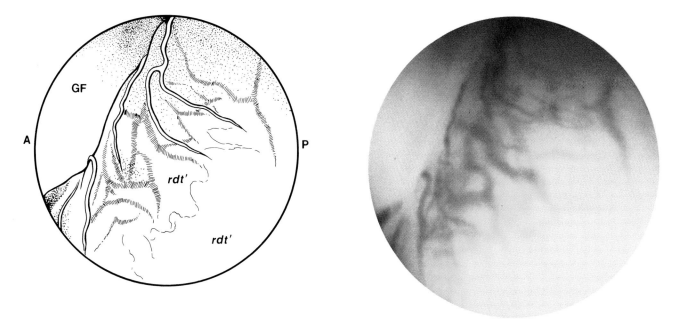

PLATE 29.   Disc Displacement Without Reduction.   Left TMJ.   Transverse Phase; Middle-central (M_c) Field.

Light is reflected off the glenoid fossa (GF) back toward the telescope to transilluminate the remodeled retrodiscal tissue (*rdt'*). The transversely oriented superficial and deep vessels are demonstrated. (**A** = anterior. **P** = posterior.)

89

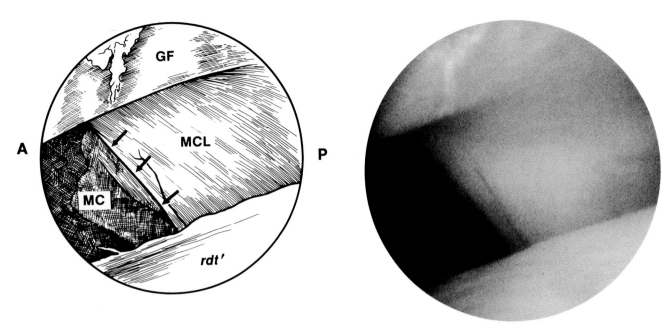

PLATE 30.   Disc Displacement Without Reduction.   Left TMJ.   Transverse Phase; Middle-central (M$_c$) Field.

The termination (arrows) of the medial capsular ligament (MCL) is apparent. The dark space anterior to the ligament is a shadow over the medial capsule (MC). Note the orientation of the fibers of the medial capsular ligament, posteroinferior to anterosuperior. A synovial blood vessel is seen coursing along this structure near its anterior margin. The glenoid fossa (GF) and remodeled retrodiscal tissue (*rdt'*) are noted. The operator may mistakenly identify remodeled retrodiscal tissue as disc, if a detailed examination is not performed. The remodeled retrodiscal tissue appears fibrillated. Note the surface irregularities, especially to the left of the field. The debris on the glenoid fossa may represent torn synovium. (**A** = anterior. **P** = posterior.)

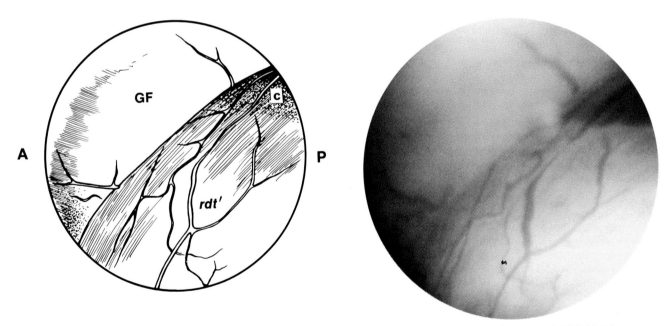

PLATE 31.   Disc Displacement With Reduction.   Left TMJ.   Transverse Phase; Middle-central (M$_c$) Field.

Note the remodeled retrodiscal tissue (*rdt'*). In the background, synovial vessels in the glenoid fossa (GF) may be seen. The vessels within the remodeled retrodiscal tissue have a generally transverse orientation. Note how the color of the remodeled retrodiscal tissue varies from ivory to dull white. The fibrous nature of this structure is distinctive. A blood clot (c), adherent to the remodeled retrodiscal tissue, is seen at the extreme right of the field. (**A** = anterior. **P** = posterior.)

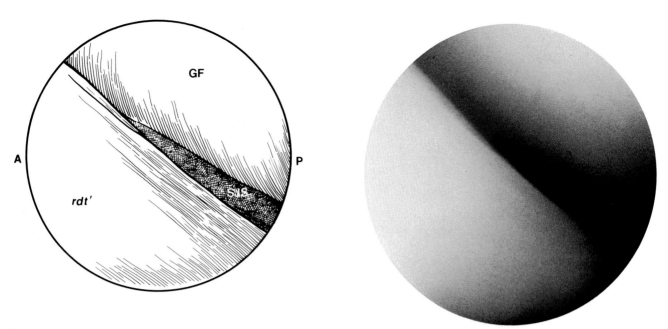

PLATE 32. Disc Displacement Without Reduction. Left TMJ. Transverse Phase; Middle-lateral (M$_l$) Field.

Extreme remodeling of the retrodiscal tissue (*rdt'*) has occurred, as demonstrated by the lack of superficial vascularity. The yellow-white color of this structure approximates that of the fibrous connective tissue–lined glenoid fossa (GF). The superior joint space (SJS) is seen to the left of the field. (**A** = anterior. **P** = posterior.)

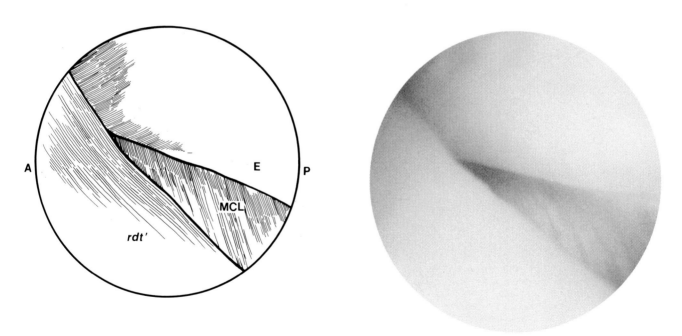

PLATE 33. Disc Displacement Without Reduction. Left TMJ. Transverse Phase; Anterior-central (A$_c$) Field.

The telescope is positioned in the anterior glenoid region. No superficial vessels are noted. Superiorly, the posterior slope of the eminence (E) can be seen. The fibrillated, remodeled retrodiscal tissue (*rdt'*) lies inferiorly. The subtle irregularities in the tissue below are signs of remodeling. The lack of a color disparity between the two tissues is an indication that the tissue below is remodeled retrodiscal tissue and not disc. Disc would appear stark white. No superficial vessels are present to assist in the diagnosis. The posteroinferior to anterosuperior orientation of the fibers of the medial capsular ligament (MCL) is seen in the background. (**A** = anterior. **P** = posterior.)

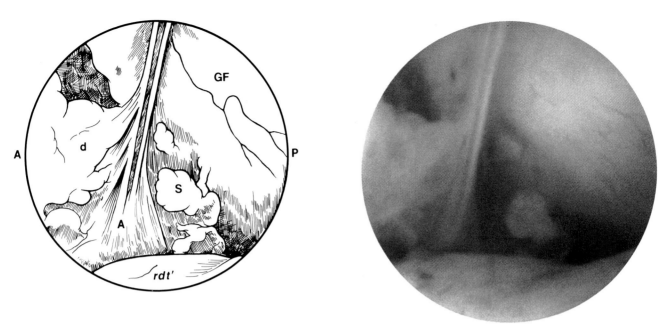

PLATE 34. Disc Displacement Without Reduction. Left TMJ. Transverse Phase; Anterior-central (A$_c$) Field.

A moderate amount of debris (d) is noted in the anterior glenoid region. A fibrous adhesive band (A) extends anteroinferiorly from the roof of the synovium–lined glenoid fossa (GF) above, to the remodeled retrodiscal tissue (*rdt'*) below. A clump of amorphous white debris to the left of the field appears connected to the adhesion. Medial and inferior to the adhesion is a small mass of yellow tissue probably representing synovium (S) that was iatrogenically stripped from the glenoid fossa. To the extreme right of the field, small-caliber synovial vessels of the glenoid fossa are visible. A small superficial vessel is noted on the remodeled retrodiscal tissue. (**A** = anterior. **P** = posterior.)

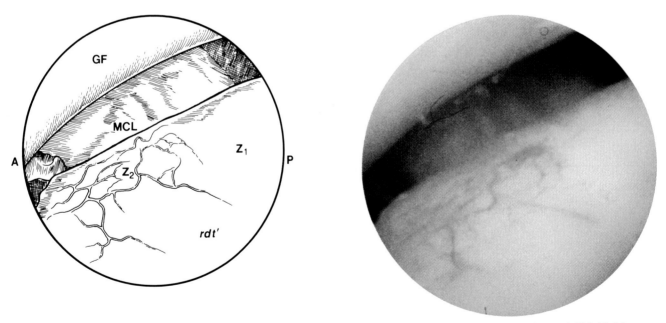

PLATE 35. Disc Displacement Without Reduction. Left TMJ. Transverse Phase; Anterior-lateral (A$_l$) Field.

Remodeled retrodiscal tissue (*rdt'*) is noted demonstrating two distinct zones: anteriorly, a zone with superficial vessels (Z$_2$), and posteriorly, an avascular zone (Z$_1$). In the dynamic transverse phase the condyle appeared to exert pressure upward on the posterior zone (Z$_1$). Above, the lateral aspect of the fibrous connective tissue–lined glenoid fossa (GF) is visible. Synovial vessels are absent. The obliquely oriented gray fibers of the medial capsular ligament (MCL) are seen in the background. (**A** = anterior. **P** = posterior.)

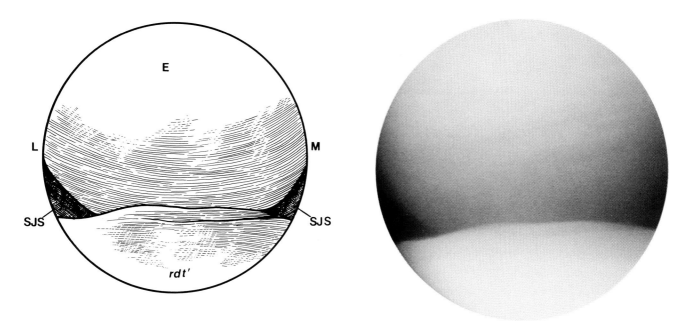

PLATE 36.   Disc Displacement Without Reduction.   Left TMJ.   Longitudinal Phase; Central (C) Field.

The remodeled retrodiscal tissue (*rdt'*) lacks any superficial vascularity and thus may easily be confused with normal disc. The color of this tissue is similar to the yellow-white of the eminence (E). In a normal condyle-disc-fossa relationship, the stark white of the disc generally contrasts sharply with the yellow-white of the coverings of the eminence and glenoid fossa. No synovial vessels are noted in this plate, as is often the case with extreme remodeling of the retrodiscal tissue. Closer inspection reveals the surface irregularities and fibrillations typical of advanced remodeling of retrodiscal tissue. Additionally, note the mismatching (lack of parallelism) of the curvatures of the remodeled retrodiscal tissue and the eminence. As a result, the superior joint space (SJS) takes on an hourglass configuration. (**L** = lateral. **M** = medial.)

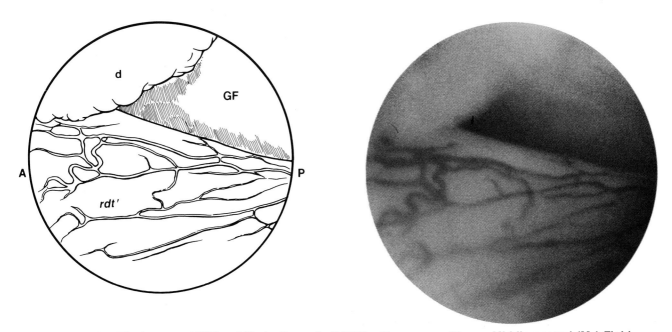

PLATE 37.   Disc Displacement Without Reduction.   Left TMJ.   Transverse Phase; Middle-central (Mc) Field.

Note the generally transverse course of the superficial vessels in the remodeled retrodiscal tissue (*rdt'*). Many anastomosing vessels are present. Some debris (d) is present in the upper left quadrant, partially obscuring the field of view. No vessels are apparent on the fibrous connective tissue–lined glenoid fossa (GF). (**A** = anterior. **P** = posterior.)

93

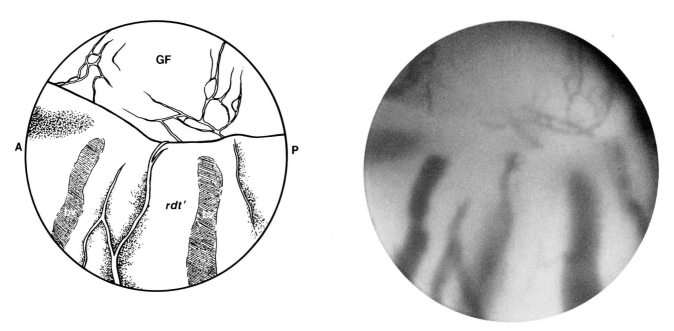

PLATE 38.   Disc Displacement Without Reduction.   Left TMJ.   Transverse Phase; Middle-central (M_c) Field.

The transverse orientation of the superficial vessels of the remodeled retrodiscal tissue (*rdt′*) is apparent. Two large-caliber blood vessels (bv) flank two vessels of smaller caliber. In the background, the inferosuperior orientation of some vessels within the synovium of the glenoid fossa (GF) is noted. Closer examination with the telescope would reveal the disparity in size between vessels of the synovium and those of the remodeled retrodiscal tissue. The small black demilune to the right of the arthroscopic field on the color plate resulted from bending of the telescope, which interrupted the transmission of light. (**A** = anterior. **P** = posterior.)

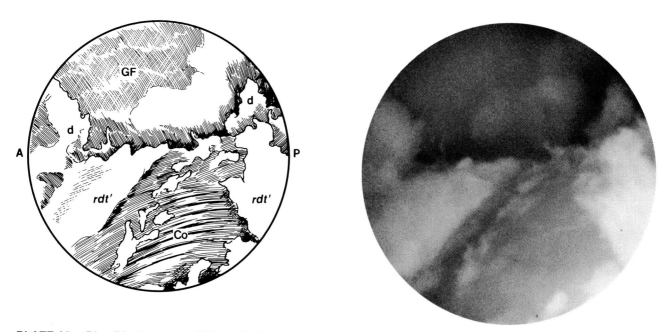

PLATE 39.   Disc Displacement Without Reduction.   Left TMJ.   Transverse Phase; Middle-central (M_c) Field.

A large perforation is located in the remodeled retrodiscal tissue (*rdt′*). No superficial vessels are noted in the fibrous connective tissue–lined glenoid fossa (GF) or in the remodeled retrodiscal tissue. The edges of the perforation are frayed. The bony surface of the condyle (Co) is roughened and appears denuded of fibrous connective tissue or cartilage. Some debris (d) is seen floating within the superior joint space. The frayed edges and floating debris suggest a traumatic tear of the thin remodeled retrodiscal tissue. The tissue adherent to the condyle, between the edges of the perforation, may represent remnants of the remodeled retrodiscal tissue or the remains of fibrous connective tissue or articular cartilage. (**A** = anterior. **P** = posterior.)

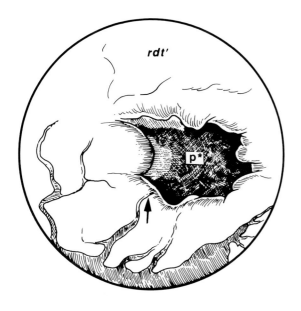

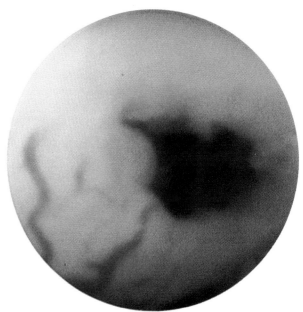

PLATE 40.   Disc Displacement Without Reduction.   Left TMJ.   Transverse Phase; Viewed Directly Over Superior Surface of the Retrodiscal Tissue.

A perforation (p∗) with irregular frayed margins is visible here. A complete examination of the superior joint space revealed that the perforation was located in the lateral portion of the remodeled retrodiscal tissue (*rdt'*). Superficial vessels are noted only to the left of the field, peripheral to the perforation. One of these vessels (arrow) appears to curl inferiorly around the edge of the perforation. The condyle, not seen here, is located beneath the perforation.

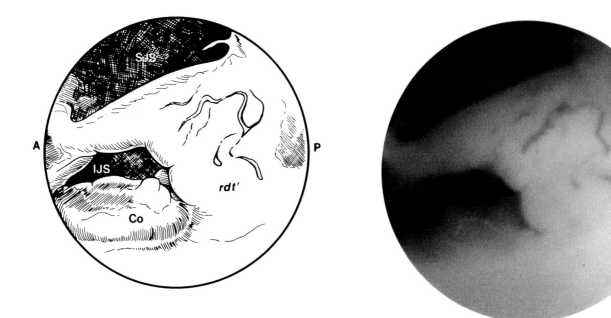

PLATE 41.   Disc Displacement Without Reduction.   Left TMJ.   Transverse Phase; Posterior-central (P_c) Field.

A perforation of the remodeled retrodiscal tissue (*rdt'*) is seen. Posteriorly, a small number of superficial vessels are noted. The orientation of these vessels is difficult to appreciate. The superior joint space (SJS) is seen above, and the inferior joint space (IJS) below. Note the granulation tissue covering the condyle (Co) below. (**A** = anterior. **P** = posterior.)

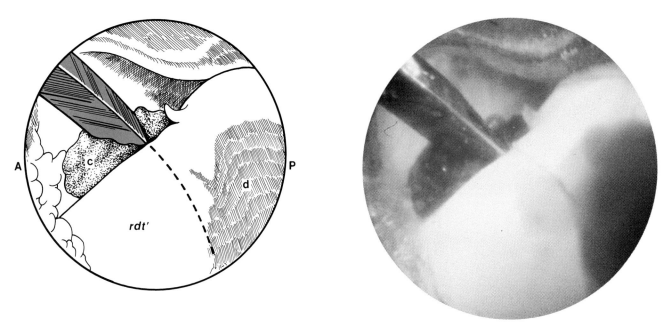

PLATE 42.   Disc Displacement Without Reduction.   Left TMJ.   Transverse Phase; Middle-central (M$_c$) Field.   Cold Retrodiscotomy Procedure.

A pediatric uretherotome seen through a 0° 2.7-mm forward viewing rod lens telescope is being used to make a releasing incision in the remodeled retrodiscal tissue (*rdt'*). A transverse releasing incision permits further disc displacement and additional remodeling of the retrodiscal tissues. A blood clot (c) is trapped behind the cutting knife. There is some debris (d) in the foreground, to the right of the field. (**A** = anterior. **P** = posterior.)

PLATES 43 to 45.   Disc Displacement With Reduction.   Left TMJ.   Transverse Phase; Middle-central (M$_c$) Field.

A transverse retrodiscotomy is being performed to separate the fibrosed remodeled retrodiscal tissue into anterior and posterior segments. See specific plate descriptions, below.

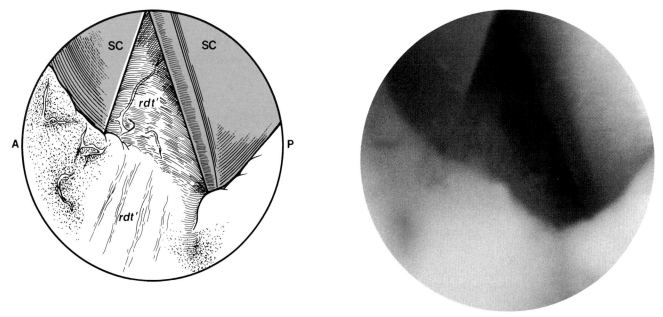

PLATE 43

A microscissors (SC) is inserted through the remodeled retrodiscal tissue (*rdt'*) to reach the inferior joint space. The blades of this particular scissors will cut tissue during both opening and closing. The incision is made in the least vascular region of the remodeled retrodiscal tissue. Note the few superficial transverse vessels to the extreme left of the field. (**A** = anterior. **P** = posterior.)

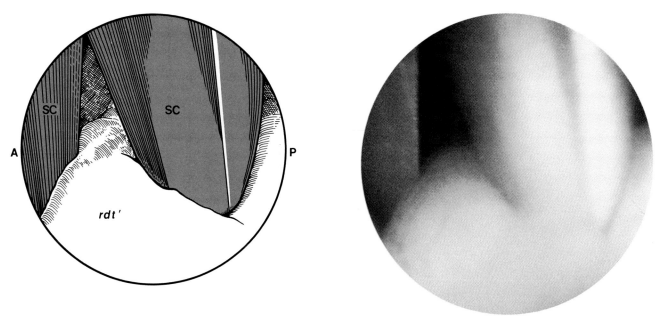

PLATE 44

The remodeled retrodiscal tissue (*rdt'*) is pinched between the blades of a microscissors (SC) to allow access to the inferior joint space. (**A** = anterior. **P** = posterior.)

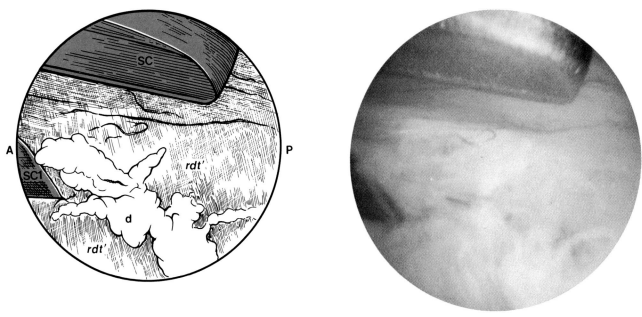

PLATE 45

The lower beak of the microscissors (SC1) has partially penetrated the remodeled retrodiscal tissue (*rdt'*); (upper beak, SC). The debris (d) created from the transection may be suctioned periodically using a suction tip. (**A** = anterior. **P** = posterior.)

PROBLEM SOLVING

COMMON PROBLEMS AND SOLUTIONS

Plates 46 to 55 found at the end of the chapter are referred to in the text. Common problems and their solutions are listed below.

PROBLEM	SOLUTION
1. A black demilune is present across the field. (Plate 46)	1. Light transmission is being interrupted owing to excessive torque on the endoscope. Release the instrument and allow it to find a passive position.
2. A brown demilune is present across the field.	2. The inside of the sheath is being viewed. Check that the telescope is properly locked to the sheath.
3. Dark, poorly defined field of view (Plate 47).	3. Irreparable damage has occurred to the rod lens telescope. Contact manufacturer's representative prior to discarding.
4. The image is sharply clearer in one area of the field of view.	4. An air bubble may be adhering to the objective lens. The image appears distorted. Clear the joint space of air bubbles by first eliminating air bubbles contained in the irrigant, and then flushing the joint space. If air bubbles persist, gently touch the telescope to nearby tissue to displace the air. Air bubbles will eventually absorb or disperse.
5. The operator is unable to identify the joint space (Plates 48, 49, 50 and 51)	5. Check that the irrigation stopcock is open. Check that the light source is functioning properly and that all fiberoptic cable connections are secured. Suction or flush the joint space to remove debris. Consider removing the external sheath/telescope and reintroducing the trocar/external sheath.

PROBLEM	SOLUTION
6. The operator is unable to negotiate the pre-eminence region.	6. Position the sheath in the anterolateral (A_1) field and then direct the blunt trocar-sheath unit anteromedially around the apex of the eminence. In many cases, the laxity of the ligaments permits entrance into the pre-eminence region without the need for posterior distraction of the condyle or removal of the telescope.
7. The image is partially obscured by tissue covering the telescope. (Plates 46 and 52)	7. Free or attached extracaspular debris may be caught on the end of the telescope. Negotiation around the attached debris is difficult because the image seen is 30 degrees off the optical axis. Usually, the telescope and sheath must be removed as a unit and a sheath and trocar reintroduced. If the debris is free, the telescope can gently be brought into contact with an intracapsular structure, such as remodeled retrodiscal tissue, to brush the debris away.
8. The operator is unable to penetrate the superior joint space with the trocar and sheath.	8. Repeat the technique for negotiating around the lateral lip of the glenoid fossa with the 19-gauge needle. On rare occasions, the needle may not be able to penetrate the superior joint space because of the inferior projection of the lateral rim of the glenoid fossa.
9. Intracapsular bleeding is present.	9. The wide angle telescopic lens and innate magnification exaggerates the appearance of bleeding. Increasing irrigation and dilation will seal the bleeding vessels.
10. Extracapsular bleeding is present.	10. Profuse extracapsular bleeding may occur owing to tearing of a branch of the superficial temporal vessels crossing the lateral capsule. Application of pressure above and below the puncture site will temporarily stop the hemorrhage. Undermine the puncture stab wound and insert, blindly, a minihemostatic clip. Bleeding may also occur from violation of the medial capsule/ligament (see below).
11. Profuse intracapsular bleeding is present.	11. Ascertaining the origin of the hemorrhage is difficult because increasing the flow of irrigation does not clear the joint space. Withdraw the telescope and apply pressure. Possible sources of bleeding include rupture of a major vessel medial to temporomandibular joint or violation of the glenoid fossa (Figs. 7-1, 7-2, 7-3). In addition, check the external auditory canal for an iatrogenic perforation. Obtain appropriate consultation.
12. Bleeding from the external auditory canal is present (Figs. 7-2, 7-3A and 7-3B)	12. Stop procedure. Iatrogenic perforation of external auditory canal is likely. Obtain immediate appropriate consultation.
13. Perforation of the medial capsular ligament (Plates 53, 54 and 55)	13. The perforation is of little significance unless bleeding occurs.

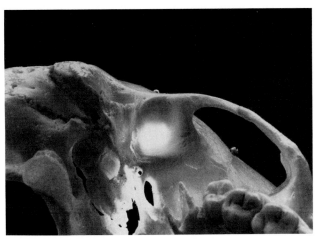

FIG. 7-1. Right TMJ, glenoid fossa seen from the infero-superior direction. The glenoid fossa has been transilluminated from above to demonstrate the thinness of the bone in this area.

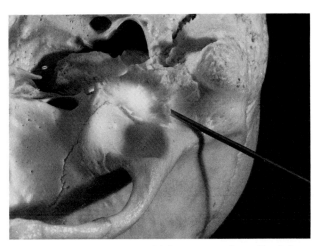

FIG. 7-2. Right TMJ, glenoid fossa seen from the infero-superior direction. The external auditory canal has been transilluminated to illustrate the thinness of the tympanic plate of the temporal bone. A dehiscence in the bony skeleton may exist here as a result of the failure of the foramen of Huschke to close during growth and development.

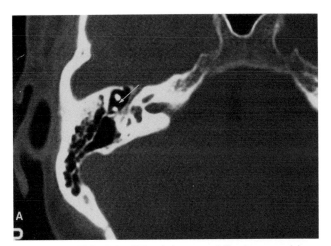

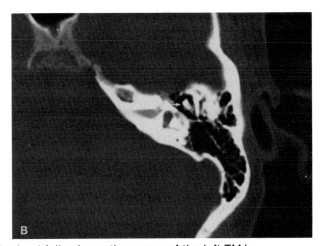

FIG. 7-3. CT axial scan of the temporal bone obtained following arthroscopy of the left TMJ. Deafness was reportedly noted immediately postoperatively. *A*, Note the complete incomalleolar dislocation (arrow). *B*, Note the normal incomalleolar relationship (arrow).

SUGGESTED READINGS

Blaustein DI, Heffez L: Diagnostic arthroscopy of the temporomandibular joint. Part 11: Pathological arthroscopic findings. Oral Surg 66(2):135–141, 1988.

Heffez L, Blaustein DI: Diagnostic arthroscopy of the temporomandibular joint. Part 1: Normal arthroscopic findings. Oral Surg 64(6):653–678, 1987

Westesson PL, Eriksson L, Liedberg J: The risk of damage to facial nerve, superficial temporal vessels, disk, and articular surfaces during arthroscopic examination of the TMJ. Oral Surg 62(2):124–7, 1986.

Van Sickels JE, Nishioka GJ, Hegewald MB, et al. Middle ear injury resulting from temporomandibular joint arthroscopy. J Oral Maxillofac Surg 45:962–965, 1987.

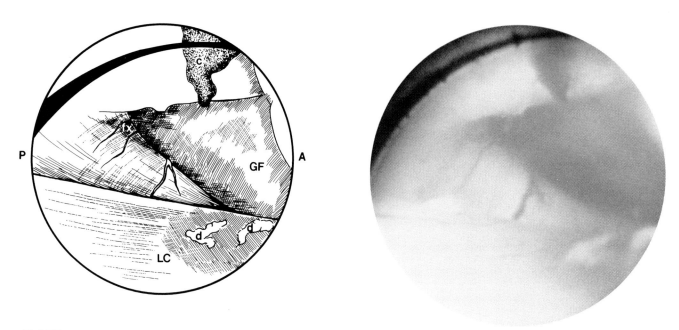

PLATE 46. Incomplete Penetration of the Superior Joint Space and Bending of the Rod Lens Telescope.   Disc Displacement With Reduction.   Right TMJ.   Transverse Phase; Posterior-lateral (P$_l$) Field.

The flexure (fx) is partly obscured inferiorly by the lateral capsule (LC). Superiorly and to the left a black crescent indicates bending of the rod lens telescope. Whenever this occurs, the operator should immediately release tension to prevent damage to the lens system. The lateral capsule is impinging on the telescope. Care should be taken not to confuse the lateral capsule with an adhesion. The telescope should be removed, the blunt trocar inserted, and the outer sheath directed more centrally. Direct manipulation of the telescope without first using the trocar would probably fail or introduce extracapsular debris. Note a clot (c) in the superior aspect of the field, debris (d) on the lateral capsule, and the glenoid fossa (GF) in the background. (**P** = posterior. **A** = anterior.)

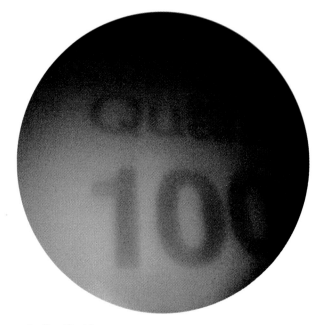

PLATE 47.   Irreparable Damage to the Rod Lens

Note the black demilune interfering with the field of vision. The demilune does not have a well-defined border, as in Plate 49. Permanent damage has been done to the rod lenses within the telescope.

102

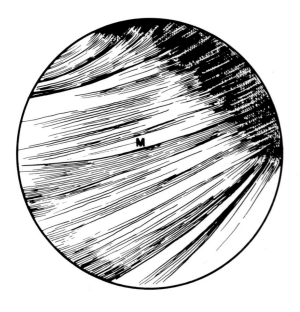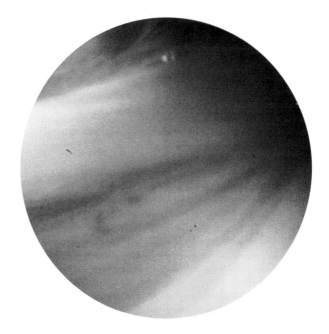

PLATE 48. External Pterygoid Muscle Fibers.

The telescope has been misdirected anteromedially and has violated the integrity of the medial capsule. No joint space is appreciated. The horizontally oriented external pterygoid muscle fibers (M) are visible.

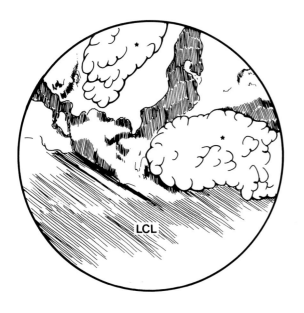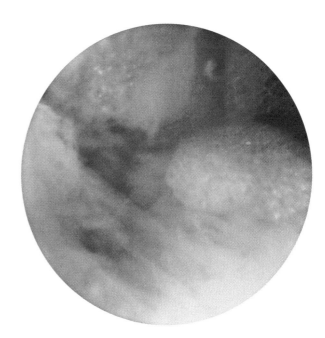

PLATE 49. Extracapsular Location of Telescope.

The telescope has slipped laterally during examination of the lateral fields of the glenoid region. It is now located immediately lateral to the lateral capsular ligament (LCL). The tissue with a golden soap-bubble appearance (*) represents either fat or parotid gland. This debris may be introduced into the joint cavity during re-entry of the trocar.

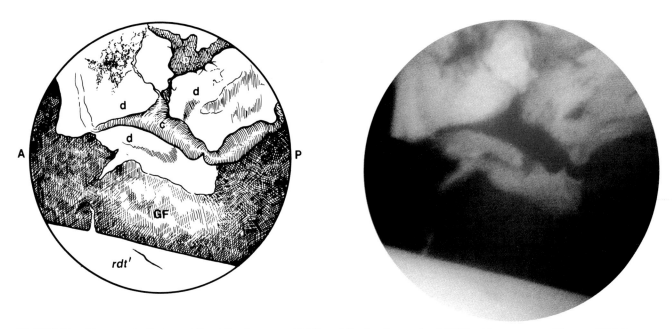

PLATE 50. Traumatic Entry. Disc Displacement Without Reduction. Left TMJ. Transverse Phase; Middle-central (M$_c$) Field.

Remodeled retrodiscal tissue (*rdt'*) demonstrating a superficial vessel is noted. A large clot (c) is visible in the center of the field. The debris (d) is synovium that has been stripped from the glenoid fossa (GF), exposing a small area of bone (b). Because of the lateral positioning of the telescope, the remainder of the synovium of the glenoid fossa is inadequately illuminated. (**A** = anterior. **P** = posterior.)

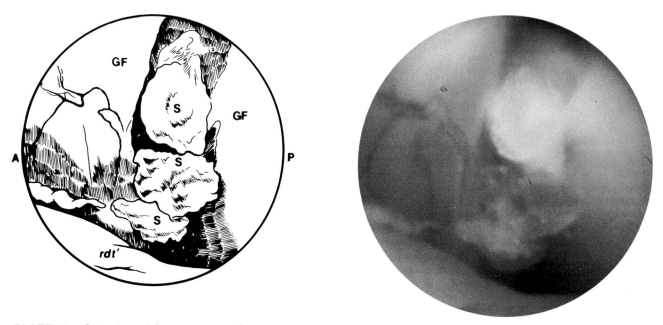

PLATE 51. Stripping of Glenoid Fossa Synovium. Disc Displacement. Left TMJ. Transverse Phase; Anterior-lateral (A$_l$) Field.

The sharp trocar has stripped the synovium (S) lining the glenoid fossa (GF), exposing the underlying bone (b). Small-caliber vessels course through the intact synovium, to the left of the field. The remodeled retrodiscal tissue (*rdt'*) is seen inferiorly. Note that the surface of this structure is irregular. (**A** = anterior. **P** = posterior.)

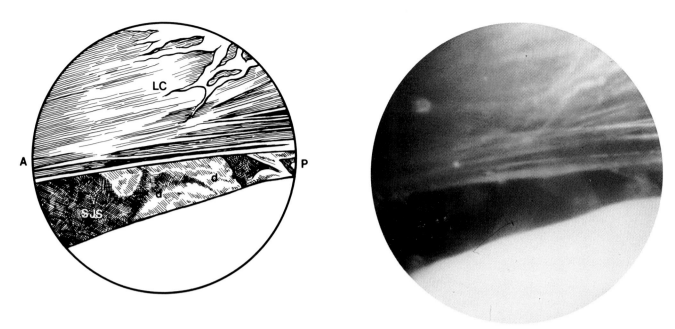

PLATE 52.   Incomplete Penetration of the Superior Joint Space.   Disc Displacement Without Reduction.   Left TMJ.   Transverse Phase; Middle-lateral (M$_l$) Field.

The superior aspect of the field is obstructed by a horizontally oriented fibrous connective tissue band. This tissue represents the lateral capsule (LC). The telescope has not completely penetrated the superior joint space (SJS). To correct this problem, the trocar should be reinserted into the sheath and directed toward the greatest concavity of the glenoid fossa. The color and nature of the disc tissue below is difficult to ascertain because of flash reflection. The background suggests the presence of debris (d) in the superior joint space. (**A** = anterior. **P** = posterior.)

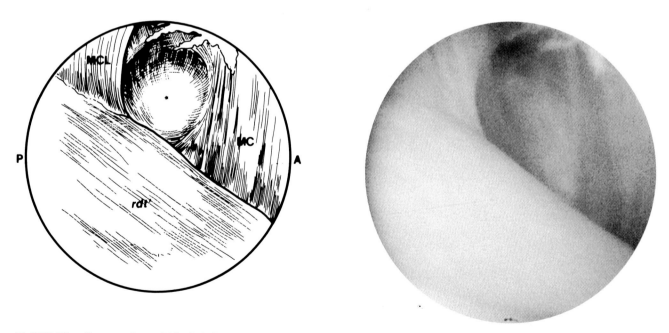

PLATE 53.   Depression of Medial Capsule.   Disc Displacement Without Reduction.   Right TMJ.   Transverse Phase; Middle-medial (M$_m$) Field.

Depression (∗) of the medial capsule (MC) without frank perforation. This indentation is located immediately anterior to the termination of the medial capsular ligament (MCL). Extremely remodeled retrodiscal tissue (*rdt'*) with no superficial vessels is noted below. Debris at the top of the field may represent torn synovium. (**P** = posterior. **A** = anterior.)

105

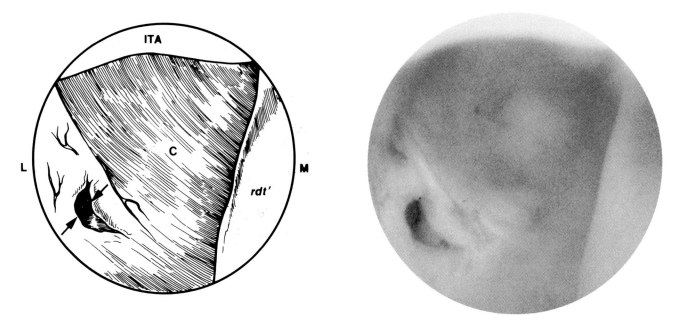

PLATE 54. Perforation of the Anterior Capsule. Disc Displacement Without Reduction. Left TMJ. Longitudinal Study; Lateral (L) Field.

The anteromedial portion of the capsule (C) is in view. An iatrogenic perforation (arrows) of the capsule may be seen. This perforation occurred during manipulation of the blunt trocar while attempting to gain access to the pre-eminence region. The ivory-colored remodeled retrodiscal tissue (*rdt'*) is to the right of the field. The infratemporal articulating surface (ITA) of the temporal bone is at the top of the field. A few vessels course in the synovium lining the capsule. (**L** = lateral. **M** = medial.)

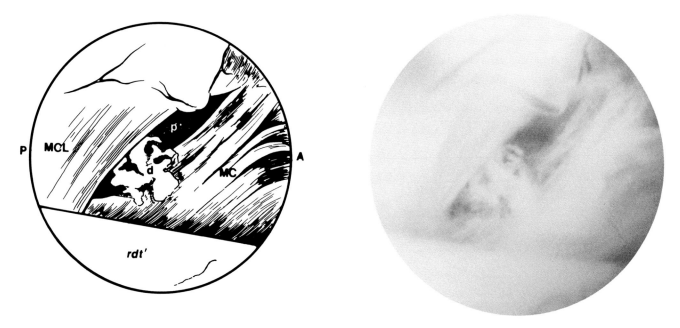

PLATE 55. Perforation of the Medial Capsule. Disc Displacement With Reduction. Right TMJ. Transverse Study; Middle-medial (M_m) Field.

There is a traumatic perforation (p*) of the medial capsule (MC), immediately anterior to the medial capsular ligament (MCL). Fluffy clouds of debris (d) have been created. Remodeled retrodiscal tissue (*rdt'*) with a single transverse vessel is seen. (**P** = posterior. **A** = anterior.)

106

adhesion: a fibrous connective tissue band fixed at both ends; an adhesion can be qualified with descriptors such as *linear* or *weblike*.

anterior incline of the posterior band: the anterior, downward slope of the posterior band of the articular disc.

contrast: a subjective appraisal of the darkest and lightest portions of the field of view.

corrugations: small surface foldings of a tissue, seen especially in the remodeled retrodiscal tissue.

crest of the posterior band: the peak of the posterior band; the junction of the posterior and anterior inclines of the posterior band.

definition: the sharpness of an image. Theoretically, an image is reproduced at the eyepiece free of optical distortion and interruptions. The fracturing of fiber threads in a flexible fiber endoscope interrupts the continuity of the image being transmitted.

depression: an interruption in the normal topography of a structure.

diameter of the telescope: the circumference of the telescope. The diameter measures the space needed to accommodate the objective lens and illuminating fibers. The diameter of the sheath that accommodates the telescope and inflow and operative channels, however, is more significant.

direction of view (angle of inclination): the angle, measured in degrees, formed between the optical system and the horizontal axis of the telescope. The direction of view bisects the viewing angle. Telescopes may have a 0, 10, 30, 70, or 120 degree direction of view to increase the viewing angle without creating any distortion. Specific directions of view vary among manufacturers.

disc (discus articularis): Stedman's defines disc as "a

plate or ring of fibrocartilage attached to the joint capsule and separating the articular surfaces of the bone for a varying distance, sometimes completely; it serves to adapt two articular surfaces that are not entirely congruent." The term *disc* is used in this text to describe an articular component that separates the joint cavity, even though it is not a fibrocartilaginous structure. Use of the term *meniscus* is inappropriate regarding the temporomandibular joint (see *meniscus*).

disc position: disc position may be approximated by judging the position of the posterior band in relation to the superior aspect of the condyle; in the normal condyle-disc-fossa relationship, the posterior band is located at about the 12 o'clock position. Disc position may also be approximated by judging the position of the thin zone on radiographs (intermediate zone) of the disc in relation to the condyle and eminence. In this method, tangents are drawn at the points of minimal (superior point) and maximal (anterior point) sectional curvatures of the condyle, and the center of the working surface of the condyle is located. The thin zone is located along the mechanical center of the joint, that is, along a perpendicular drawn from the center of the working surface of the condyle to the posterior slope of the eminence..

dynamic examination phase: third of the three phases of a complete diagnostic examination of the superior joint space; performed while holding the telescope stationary in the approximate transverse axis of the space and manipulating the condyle downward and forward.

fiberscope: a flexible endoscope in which both the transmitting and illuminating mechanisms are glass fibers. The specific arrangement of the transmitting fibers at the working end is maintained up to the eyepiece (coherence of fiber bundles) to prevent scrambling and distortion of the image.

fibrillated: description of a structure when its surface appears composed of individual fibrils.

field of view (field of vision): a conical area determined by the viewing angle. The apex of the cone is the objective lens of the telescope.

flexure: in the normal condyle-disc-fossa relationship, the junction of the tympanic portion of the retrodiscal tissue with the posterior incline of the posterior band. In the displaced disc, the flexure is formed by the junction of the tympanic portion of the retrodiscal tissue and the remodeled retrodiscal tissue.

glenoid region: that part of the superior space located under the glenoid fossa; the region is bounded posteriorly by the attachment of the tympanic portion of the retrodiscal tissue and anteriorly by the apex of the eminence. The glenoid region is divided into *anterior* and *posterior glenoid regions* by an imaginary vertical plane dropped from the area of maximum concavity of the glenoid fossa. To record fields of view, the glenoid region is divided into a grid by the intersection of three transverse regions (anterior, posterior, middle) and three parasagittal regions (lateral, central, medial). Each of the nine arthroscopic fields thus formed may be located by describing a transverse-parasagittal coordinate.

lateral fold (pleat): a laterally located, thickened, cordlike structure within the tympanic portion of the retrodiscal tissue.

lateral sulcus (lateral paradiscal groove): the groove formed by the reflection of the lateral capsule onto the lateral edge of the disc.

light transmission: the efficiency by which an instrument is capable of transmitting light to the naked eye.

longitudinal examination phase: second of the three phases of a complete examination of the superior joint space; performed with the telescope approximating the longitudinal (sagittal) axis of the space; examination of the pre-eminence region.

magnification: the size of the image. This parameter depends on the design of the optical components. The viewing angle, ocular enlargements, and object-lens distance all influence the magnification.

medial fold (pleat): a medially thickened, cordlike structure within the tympanic portion of the retrodiscal tissue.

medial sulcus (medial paradiscal synovial groove): the groove formed by the reflection of the medial capsule onto the mediosuperior edge of the disc;

meniscus: an internal, crescent-shaped firbrocarti-lage. The term should not be applied to the temporomandibular joint.

posterior incline of the posterior band: the posterior, upward slope of the posterior band of the articular disc.

pre-eminence region: represents that portion of the superior joint space bounded posteriorly by the apex of the eminence and anteriorly by the anterior and anteromedial capsule. Fields of view, recorded lateromedially, are *lateral, central,* and *medial.*

remodeled posterior band: a posterior band altered in both shape and internal fiber architectural pattern.

remodeled retrodiscal tissue: used synonomously with remodeled posterior attachment.

resolution: the ability to discriminate as two separate images, two objects separated by the smallest distance *d.*

rigid endoscope: an inflexible endoscope with a series of incoherent glass fibers (lack of specific bundle arrangement) as the illuminating mechanism and a series of lenses as the transmitting mechanism. One exception is the selfoscope lens system. The arthroscope is an example of a rigid endoscope

synovial plicae: the smooth reflections or folds of the capsule lining. A prominent plica is often located in the Posterior-medial field.

transverse examination phase: first of the three phases of a complete diagnostic examination of the superior joint space; performed with the telescope approximating the transverse plane of the space to examine the glenoid region.

triangulation: the technique by which the telescope and instrument/suction are manipulated separately from outside the joint space to directly visualize the instrument or allow continuous outflow of irrigant. The term has also been used to describe the manipulation of three instruments in a joint space. The term *biangulation* is used in this case to describe the manipulation of two instruments.

viewing angle: the measurement that determines the diameter of the field of view. The boundaries are the outer limits at which portions of an object(s) are perceived.

virtual field: the diameter of the field as perceived through the eyepiece of the telescope. The virtual field is constant for the instrument and unrelated to the object-lens distance. To assess the virtual field, look at a series of circles of various diameters placed at an optimum distance from your eye, and simultaneously look through the telescope and try to match the diameter of the telescopic image with the diameter of the real image.

IMPORTANT DATES IN ENDOSCOPY AND ARTHROSCOPY*

1806   Bozzini used a wax candle mounted in a tin tube to facilitate the examination of deeply located organs.

1867   Desormeaux described a means of examining the genitourinary passages using an open tube endoscope. He developed the idea of a light source using a small flame burning a mixture of alcohol and turpentine. He realized the importance of a lens system to concentrate the beam of light.

1868   Bevan identified esophageal strictures and extracted foreign bodies using a 4-inch long, ¾-inch wide tube with candlelight as the light source.

1870   Waldenburg improved Bevan's technique by developing a longer instrument in which two silver tubes were "telescoped" within each other. One of the tubes carried the light source.

1870   Kussmaul performed esophagogastroscopy on a professional sword swallower, proving that a rigid tube could be used to examine the digestive tract.

1879   Nitze collaborated with Beneche, an optician, and Leiter, an instrument maker, to design the first cystoscope. The cystoscope had an outside diameter of 7 mm and a prism as the optical system. A burning platinum wire was used as the light source.

1881   Mikulicz, with Leiter, introduced a gastroscope.

1882   Nitze developed the first successful photographic endoscope. Later published his *Cystophotographic Atlas* (1884).

1887   Nitze introduced an electric globe as the light source.

1887   Stoerk developed the first remote-control mechanism for an esophagoscope, similar to the Waldenburg model.

1895   Rosenheim introduced flexible rubber obturators for safer endoscopy.

1897   Kelling employed a flexible scope that could be stiffened and thus straightened as needed.

1898   Killian attempted bronchoscopy using cocaine as a local anesthetic. He is known as the father of bronchoscopy.

1918   Takagi used a cystoscope to examine a tubercular knee.

1920   Takagi developed his first arthroscope, a 7.3-mm instrument patterned after the Charrier No. 22 cystoscope.

1921   Bircher proposed gas arthroscopy of the knee using oxygen or carbon dioxide and a Jacobeus laparascope.

1925   First report of arthroscopy in the American literature. Kreuscher reported the diagnosis of meniscal disorders.

1931   Finkelstein and Mayer performed punch biopsies of the knee under arthroscopic control.

1931   Burman reported the results of arthroscopic examination of the ankle, elbow, hip, knee, shoulder, and wrist joints. He carried out investigations into the results of vital staining of articular cartilage.

1931   Takagi developed a 3.5-mm arthoscope suitable for examination of smaller joints when saline dilation was used.

---

* Dates indicated in bold pertain specifically to the development of temporomandibular joint arthroscopy.

1932 Takagi produced the first black-and-white arthroscopic photographs.

1934 Burman, Finkelstein, and Mayer commented on the accuracy of the arthroscopic diagnosis of meniscal disorders.

1936 Takagi produced the first arthroscopic color pictures and moving pictures.

1940 Miki performed arthroscopy on the dog and found that normal saline solution at 33° and 35°C and pressure of 50 to 70 cm H_2O was the most suitable medium for joint dilation.

1955 Watanabe performed first knee arthroscopic surgery to remove a giant cell tumor.

1957 Watanabe obtained photographs by coupling a 35-mm camera system to his No. 21 arthroscope. The No. 19 telescope was used for routine examination.

1957 First *Atlas of Arthroscopy* was published by Watanabe, a student of Takagi.

1955–1959 Takagi, Watanabe, Takeda, and Ikeuchi developed single-puncture and multiple-puncture (triangulation) techniques. The Watanabe Type #21 arthroscope was developed. These clinicians performed arthroscopic synovial biopsies, cautery of intra-articular structures, extraction of loose bodies, resection of tumors, partial meniscectomies, and total excision of lateral menisci. Modern arthroscopy was thus born.

1960 Hopkins introduced the rod lens endoscopic system.

1965 Jackson, an orthopedic surgeon, began teaching arthroscopy in Toronto, Canada after being taught the technique by Watanabe, Ikeuchi, and Takeda in Tokyo.

1967 Fiberoptic light system was invented.

1970 Watanabe #24 Selfoc arthroscope (1.7-mm diameter, 2-mm sheath) was distributed in the United States under the brand name Needlescope (Dyonics Company).

1970 Ohnishi reported on arthroscopy of the cadaver temporomandibular joint.

1972 Jackson and Abe reported their experience in 200 cases using the #21 Watanabe arthroscope.

1974 International Arthroscopy Association was founded.

1975 The first report of diagnostic TMJ arthroscopy was made by Ohnishi, 57 years after the earliest attempt at knee arthroscopy.

1975 American Academy of Orthopedic Surgeons sponsored instructional courses.

1976 First North American arthroscopic textbook was published *Arthroscopy of the Knee* by Jackson and Dandy.

1978 O'Connor established first course on operative arthroscopy of the knee.

1978 Hilsabeck and Laskin reported on arthroscopy of the rabbit TMJ.

1980 Williams and Laskin reported on the arthroscopic appearance of experimentally induced conditions of the rabbit TMJ.

1985 Holmlund and Hellsing described soft-tissue landmarks for arthroscopic TMJ penetration.

1986 First International Symposium on Arthoscopy of the Temporomandibular Joint was held, New York.

1986 Sanders reported on the treatment of persistent closed lock using a blind sweeping arthoscopic technique.

1987 American Association of Oral and Maxillofacial Surgeons sponsored the first symposium on arthroscopy of the TMJ. It was held in Anaheim, California.

1987/88 Heffez and Blaustein described the arthroscopic criteria for normal TMJ disc position and internally deranged joints.

1988 American Association of Oral and Maxillofacial Surgeons sponsored a symposium on controversies in TMJ arthoscopy.

SUGGESTED READINGS

Berci G: *Endoscopy.* New York, Appleton-Century-Crofts, 1976.

Bircher E: Die Arthroendoskopie. Zentrabl Chir 48:1460, 1921.

Blaustein DI, Heffez L: Diagnostic arthroscopy of the temporomandibular joint. Part 11: Pathological arthroscopic findings. Oral Surg 66(2):135–41, 1988.

Burke R: Temporomandibular joint diagnosis: Arthroscopy. J Craniomand Pract 3:233–236, 1985.

Burman MS: Arthroscopy, the direct visualization of joints: An experimental cadaver study. J Bone Joint Surg (Am) 13(4):669, 1931.

DeHaven KE, Collins HR: Diagnosis of internal derangements of the knee: The role in arthroscopy. J Bone Joint Surg (Am) 57:802–810, 1975.

Eriksson E, Sebik A: Arthroscopy and arthroscopic surgery in a gas versus a fluid medium. Symposium on arthroscopic knee surgery. Orthop Clin No Am 13:293–298, 1982.

Miki M: Influence of the temperature and pressure of the medium on the arthroscopic findings of the blood vessels of the synovial membrane (in Japanese). J Jap Orthop Assoc 16:405–439, 1941.

Finkelstein H, Mayer L: The arthroscope: A new method of examining joints. J Bone Joint Surg (Am) 13:583, 1931.

Goss AN, Dosanquet P, Tideman H: The accuracy of temporomandibular joint arthroscopy. J Maxillofac Surg 15(2):99–102, 1987.

Heffez L, Blaustein DI: Diagnostic arthroscopy of the temporomandibular joint. Part 1: Normal arthroscopic findings. Oral Surg 64(6):653–678, 1987.

Hellsing G, Holmlund A, Nordenram A, et al. Arthroscopy of the temporomandibular joint. Examination of 2 patients with suspected disk derangement. Int J Oral Surg 13:69–74, 1984.

Hilsabeck RB, Laskin DM: Arthroscopy of the temporomandibular joint of the rabbit. J Oral Surg 36(12):938–943, 1978.

Holmlund A, Hellsing G: Arthroscopy of the temporomandibular joint. An autopsy study. Int J Oral Surg 14:169–175, 1985.

Holmlund A, Hellsing G, Wredmark T: Arthroscopy of the temporomandibular joint. A clinical study. Int J Oral Maxillofac Surg 15(6):715–21, 1986.

Jackson RW, Dandy DJ: *Arthroscopy of the Knee.* New York, Grune & Stratton, 1976.

Kino K: Morphological and structural observation of the synovial membranes and their folds relating to the endoscopic findings in the upper cavity of the human temporomandibular joint (in Japanese, English abstract). J Jap Stomat 47:98–134, 1980.

Kino K, Ohnishi M, Shioda S, et al. Morphological observation on the inner surface of the temporomandibular joint. Histological investigation relating to the arthroscopic findings in the upper cavity (in Japanese). Japan J Oral Surg 27:1379, 1981.

Kussmaul J: Über Magenspiegelung. Verh Naturforschenden Ges Freiburg 5:112, 1870.

Liedberg J, Westesson PL: Diagnostic accuracy of upper compartment arthroscopy of the temporomandibular joint. Correlation with postmortem morphology. Oral Surg 62(6):618–24, 1986.

McCain JP: Arthroscopy of the human temporomandibular joint. J Oral MaxFac Surg 46:648–655, 1988.

Murakami K et al.: Arthroscopic differential diagnoses and treatments of the locking symptoms of the temporomandibular joint and their regional anatomical interpretations. European Association for Maxillo-facial Surgery, 7th Congress Paris, France.

Murakami K, Hoshino K: Regional anatomical nomenclature and arthroscopic terminology in human tempormandibular joints. Okajimas Folla Anat Jpn 58:745–760, 1982.

Murakami K, Matsuki M, Iizuka T, et al. Diagnostic arthroscopy of the TMJ: Differential diagnoses in patients with limited jaw opening. J Craniomand Pract 4:118–126, 1986.

Murakami K, Ono T: Temporomandibular joint arthroscopy by inferolateral approach. Int J Oral Maxillofac Surg 15:410–417, 1986.

Murakami KI, Hoshino K: Histological studies on the inner surfaces of the articular cavities of human temporomandibular joints with special reference to arthroscopic observations. Anat Anz Jena 160:167–177, 1985.

Murakami KI, Matsumoto K, Iizuka T: Suppurative arthritis of the temporomandibular joint. J MaxFac Surg 12:41–45, 1984.

Nuelle D, Alpern MC, Ufema JW: Arthroscopic surgery of the temporomandibular joint. The Angle Orthodontist 56:118–141, 1986.

Ohnishi M: Arthroscopy of the temporomandibular joint (in Japanese). J Jap Stomat 42:207–213, 1975.

Ohnishi M: Clinical application of arthroscopy in the temporomandibular joint diseases. Bull Tokyo Med Dent Univ 27:141–150, 1980.

Ohnishi M: Clinical studies on the intraarticular puncture of the temporomandibular joints and its application (in Japanese). Jap J Oral Surg 22:436–442, 1970.

Ohnishi M: Diagnostic application of arthroscope to ankylosis of the temporomandibular joint (in Japanese). Jap J Oral Surg 22:436–442, 1976.

Sanders B, Buoncristiani R: Diagnostic and surgical arthroscopy of the temporomandibular joint: Clinical experience with 137 procedures over a 2 year period. J Craniomand Disorders: Facial and Oral Pain 1(3):202–213, 1987.

Sanders B: Arthroscopic surgery of temporomandibular joint:Treatment of internal derangement with persistent closed lock. Oral Surg 62:361–372, 1986.

Shahriaree H: *O'Connor's Textbook of Arthroscopic Surgery.* Philadelphia, JB Lippincott Co., 1984.

Takagi K: Practical experience using Takagi's arthroscope. J Jap Orthop Assoc 8:132, 1933.

Takagi K: The arthroscope. J Jap Orthop Assoc 14:359, 1939.

Van Sickels JE, Nishioka GJ, Hegewald MB, et al. Middle ear injury resulting from temporomandibular joint arthroscopy. J Oral Maxillofac Surg 45(11):962–965, 1987.

Watanabe M(ed): *Arthroscopy of Small Joints.* Tokyo, Igaku Shoin. 1985.

Watanabe M, Takeda S, Ikeuchi H: *Atlas of Arthroscopy*, Tokyo, Igaku Shoin, 1957.

Watanabe M, Takeda S: The Number 21 Arthroscope. J Jap Ortho Assoc 34:1041, 1960.

Watanabe M: Arthroscopic diagnosis of the internal derangements of the knee joint. J Jap Orthopaed Assoc 42:993, 1968.

Westesson PL, Eriksson L, Liedberg J: The risk of damage to facial nerve, superficial temporal vessels, disk, and articular surfaces during arthroscopic examination of the TMJ. Oral Surg 62(2):124–7, 1986.

Williams RA, Laskin DM: Arthroscopic examination of experimentally induced pathologic conditions of the rabbit temporomandibular joint. J Oral Surg 38:652–659, 1980.

INDEX

Page numbers in *italics* refer to figures and plates.